MONOGRAPHS IN
ORGANIC FUNCTIONAL GROUP ANALYSIS
GENERAL EDITORS: R. BELCHER AND D. M. W. ANDERSON

VOLUME 6

ANALYTICAL METHODS FOR ORGANIC CYANO GROUPS

OTHER TITLES IN THE SERIES IN
ORGANIC FUNCTIONAL GROUP ANALYSIS

Vol. 1. DOBINSON, HOFMANN and STARK: *The Determination of Epoxide Groups*
Vol. 2. DRYHURST: *Periodate Oxidation of Diol and Other Functional Groups: Analytical and Structural Applications*
Vol. 3. TIWARI and SHARMA: *The Determination of Carboxylic Functional Groups*
Vol. 4. JOHNSON and SIDDIQI: *The Determination of Organic Peroxides*
Vol. 5. MALONE: *The Determination of Hydrazino–Hydrazide Groups*

ANALYTICAL METHODS FOR ORGANIC CYANO GROUPS

BY

M. R. F. ASHWORTH

M.A., B.Sc. (Oxon.), Ph.D. (Aberdeen), R.N. Dr. (Prague)

Professor of Applied and Organic-Analytical Chemistry
Universität des Saarlandes, West Germany

PERGAMON PRESS

OXFORD · NEW YORK · TORONTO
SYDNEY · BRAUNSCHWEIG

Pergamon Press Ltd., Headington Hill Hall, Oxford
Pergamon Press Inc., Maxwell House, Fairview Park, Elmsford, New York 10523
Pergamon of Canada Ltd., 207 Queen's Quay West, Toronto 1
Pergamon Press (Aust.) Pty. Ltd., 19a Boundary Street, Rushcutters Bay, N.S.W. 2011, Australia
Vieweg & Sohn GmbH, Burgplatz 1, Braunschweig

First edition 1971

Library of Congress Catalog Card No. 73–137135

Printed in Great Britain by Page Brothers (Norwich) Ltd.

08 016191 X

CONTENTS

PREFACE

BOTH qualitative and quantitative analytical information are contained in this monograph.

There are several ways of classifying and presenting analytical data on a compound class: according to the type of compound; into laboratory and technical parts; chronologically; into chemical, pure physical and other (biological) methods; according to the reactions undergone (for chemical methods). The last mentioned two principles have been adopted here. This is deemed a more fundamental classification, and illustrates the relation between qualitative and quantitative principles. It means, of course, that data on important individual compounds such as acrylonitrile or cyanamide are scattered through the monograph. It is hoped that the index and cross-references will assist the reader to overcome this small inconvenience.

The contents are accordingly divided into two major parts: (A) chemical methods, classified as far as possible according to the reaction undergone by the compound being detected, identified or determined; and (B) physical methods, principally pure physical methods (polarographic procedures are grouped here, although they are in fact based on reduction).

M.R.F.A.

CHAPTER 1

INTRODUCTION

The two principal compound classes considered in this monograph are the "genuine" nitriles, containing the $-\overset{|}{\underset{|}{C}}-CN$ group, and the *N*-cyano compounds, such as cyanamide and related compounds, possessing the $-\overset{|}{N}-CN$ group. Organic thiocyanates and possible cyanates, having the —S—CN and —O—CN groups, respectively, will be discussed in a later monograph along with the corresponding iso-series, isothiocyanates and isocyanates.

Many compounds are known in which cyano groups are attached to other elements. Most are, however, ineligible for inclusion under organic cyano compounds: e.g., the familiar complex cyanides of transition metals such as iron, cobalt, and nickel. Two exceptions have been made here, namely, cyanocobalamin and the so-called nerve gas, "Tabun"; these contain a Co–CN and P–CN linkage, respectively.

Organic cyano compounds occur rarely in nature. The most important compound of this class is the anti-pernicious anaemia factor, cyanocobalamin or vitamin B_{12}. Some glucosides, such as amygdalin, also contain the cyano group and are cyanohydrins. Some nitriles have been found in small amounts in products of petroleum or coal origin. In earlier work, the carboxylic acids formed on hydrolysis generally served for identification. In this way, Kruber and Marx[1] in 1938 found α-naphthonitrile in the anthracene oil of hard coal distillates (b.p. 299–303°) and fluorene nitriles accompanying phenanthrene. Iida and Tanaka[2] identified long-chain nitriles in shale oils, and Mapstone[3] concluded that Australian shale oil contains nitriles. The later development of chromatographic methods (especially gas chromatography) for separation and identification, and of ultraviolet, infrared, and mass spectrometry for identification, has enabled this work to be extended. Thus Van Meter and co-workers[4] found benzonitrile and its 2- and 3-methyl derivatives in shale oil naphtha fractions of boiling-point up to 200°, using ultraviolet and mass spectra for identification. Sokol *et al.*[5] identified lower aliphatic nitriles in the benzene (b.p. 60–150°) from carbonisation of brown coal, using a combination of gas chromatography and infrared. Hartung and Jewell[6] showed the presence of numerous aromatic (benzene, indene, biphenyl, naphthalene) and naphthene (cyclohexane, hydrogenated naphthalenes) nitriles in hydrogenated furnace oil, identifying by means of ultraviolet and mass spectrometry. Iida *et al.*[7] found straight chain C_{12}–C_{15} nitriles (but only in 0·2% amounts) in a Colorado shale oil fraction of b.p. 280–305°, making use of infrared spectra and gas chromatography as well as chemical methods (hydrolysis to amides with sulphuric acid) for identification. (Further details about these separations and identifications are given under the relevant headings in the main text below.)

Wahlroos and Saarivirta[8] have isolated benzonitrile from green plants by steam distillation and ether extraction and identified it with the help of gas chromatography.

On the other hand, there are numerous important synthetic nitriles. Acrylonitrile comes first to mind, a monomer for synthesis of the polymer Orlon and of some synthetic rubbers. Adiponitrile is a technical starting material for preparing adipic acid and hexamethylenediamine and hence of nylon. Some lower aliphatic nitriles are useful solvents, with acetonitrile playing a significant role in many physico-chemical and analytical studies and procedures. Higher aliphatic nitriles have found use as solvents and plasticisers. Some of these higher-boiling nitriles have been introduced in recent years as liquid phases in gas chromatography. Most are 2-cyanoethylated compounds. Possibly the most prominent representative is 1,2,3-tris(2-cyanoethoxy)propane, proposed in 1961 by McNair and DeVries[9] for separating mixtures of hydrocarbons and other compound classes such as alcohols, esters, ketones, and halides. It has been subsequently used by, amongst others, Clemons *et al.*[10] for separating C_6–C_{10} aromatics having saturated and unsaturated side-chains and by Jordan,[11] in a mixture with SE-30 gum rubber, for a number of applications where hydrocarbons were involved; 1,2,6-tris(2-cyanoethoxy)hexane is a similarly useful liquid phase. Frisone[12] has recommended *N,N'*-bis(2-cyanoethyl)formamide on account of its high selectivity for polar materials. Lemoine[13] has proposed tetracyanoethylated pentaerythritol as a selective liquid phase for separation of aromatic hydrocarbons. Assmann *et al.*[14] have recently recommended poly(vinylformalpropionitrile), a polar liquid phase, stable up to 330°, for separating compound classes such as polyols and methyl esters of fatty acids. Russian investigators,[15–19] e.g. Borodulina and co-workers and Nikolaeva and co-workers, have used 2,2′-dicyanodipropyl ether and sulphide and also succinonitrile as the liquid phase in analyses of reaction mixtures from syntheses of acrylonitrile and methacrylonitrile (see also pp. 110–2). Döring and Hauthal[20] have tried out columns of numerous cyano compounds in gas chromatographic studies of C_6 hydrocarbons. As long ago as 1956, van de Craats[21] suggested the use of silver nitrate–benzyl cyanide for separation of saturated and olefinic materials based on the tendency of the last-named to form silver complexes. This principle has been extended to higher temperatures by Zlatkis *et al.*[22] using silver nitrate with less volatile nitriles, such as *m*- and *p*-xylyl cyanides, 1-naphthylacetonitrile, 3,4-dimethylphenylacetonitrile, and oleyl nitrile. Rotzsche[23] prepared cyanoalkyl substituted silicone oils and showed how polarity and hence selectivity could be changed by varying the number of nitrile groups in the molecule.

Some nitriles are useful intermediates for introducing the carboxyl group (through subsequent hydrolysis) and for ascending homologous series (Kiliani reaction). Cyanoacetic ester is used in syntheses of saturated and unsaturated carboxylic acids.

Trichloroacetonitrile is an insecticide and fumigant. Azobisisobutyronitrile and similar compounds have been proposed as polymerisation initiators based on their ready elimination of nitrogen to yield radicals.[24]

Cyanamide and dicyanodiamide are important representatives of the compound class containing the $-\overset{|}{\mathrm{N}}-\mathrm{CN}$ group. Calcium cyanamide is a well-known fertiliser and is the starting material for the synthesis of thiourea (reaction with ammonium sulphide) and of the dimer, dicyanodiamide. Melamine and guanidine salts are prepared from dicyanodiamide.

"Tabun", the ethyl ester of dimethylphosphoramidocyanidic acid, is one of the "nerve gases" which act as poisons through inhibiting the action of choline esterase. In a recent patent, an "anti-riot" material, containing an *o*-substituted (F, Cl, NO_2, CN, or OH) benzylidene-malononitrile, has been proposed.[25]

Interest in cyanohydrocarbons is increasing. These include cyanoalkanes, such as tetra- and hexacyanoethane and tricyanomethane; cyanoalkenes such as tri- and tetracyanoethylene and hexacyanobutadiene;

dicyanoacetylene; aromatic compounds such as 1,2,4,5-tetracyanobenzene (pyromellitic nitrile) and hexacyanobenzene. Non-hydrocarbons which may be included along with the compounds mentioned are: carbonyl cyanide; dicyanodiazomethane; oxiranes such as 2,2,3,3-tetracyanooxirane (tetracyanoethylene oxide) and 7,7,8,8-tetracyanoquinodimethane. These compounds have been reviewed recently by Fischer.(26) They possess extremely negative substituents and can take part in numerous new and interesting reactions. Tetracyanoethylene appears to be a key substance for synthesising many products of high cyano content. In particular, nucleophilic attack of water, amines and sulphides on it lead to heterocyclic products. Charge-transfer complexes are formed by olefines and aromatics with the strongly electron-accepting cyanohydrocarbons; some of these reactions have been adapted for quantitative determinations in recent years.(27–30) As Fischer points out, there are already indications of the practical usefulness of cyanohydrocarbons as, for example, dyes, pigments, rocket propellents, lubricants and organic semiconductors (chemistors, photo resistances and fluorescent agents). One may expect a rapid development in this field.

Summing up, it is evident that there has been, there is, and there will continue to be adequate stimulation for development of analytical methods for cyano compounds.

References

1. KRUBER, O. and MARX, A., *Chem. Ber.* **71**, 2478 (1938).
2. IIDA, T. and TANAKA, M., *J. Pharm. Soc. Japan* **64**, 33 (1944).
3. MAPSTONE, G. E., *J. and Proc. Roy. Soc. New South Wales* **82**, 85 (1948); **83**, 80 (1949).
4. VAN METER, R. A., BAILEY, C. W., SMITH, J. R., MOORE, R. T., ALLBRIGHT, C. S., JACOBSON, I. A., Jr., HYLTON, V. M., and BALL, J. S., *Anal. Chem.* **25**, 1758 (1952).
5. SOKOL, L., KVAPIL, Z., and KARAS, V., *Coll. Czech. Chem. Commun.* **26**, 2278 (1961).
6. HARTUNG, G. K. and JEWELL, D. M., *Anal. Chim. Acta* **27**, 219 (1962).
7. IIDA, T., YOSHI, E., and KITATSUJI, E., *Anal. Chem.* **38**, 1224 (1966).
8. WAHLROOS, Ö. and SAARIVIRTA, M., *Acta Chem. Scand.* **18**, 2191 (1964).
9. MCNAIR, H. M. and DEVRIES, T., *Anal. Chem.* **33**, 806 (1961).
10. CLEMONS, C. A., LEACH, P. W., and ALTSHULLER, A. P., *Anal. Chem.* **35**, 1546 (1963).
11. JORDAN, J. H., *J. Gas Chromatog.* **2**, 346 (1964).
12. FRISONE, G. J., *Nature (London)* **193**, 370 (1962).
13. LEMOINE, T. J., *J. Gas Chromatog.* **3**, 322 (1965).
14. ASSMANN, K., SERFAS, O., and GEPPERT, G., *J. Chromatog.* **26**, 495 (1967).
15. BORODULINA, R. I., VERTEBNI, P. YA., and REVEL'SKII, I. A., *Gazov Khromatogr., Akad. Nauk SSSR, Tr. Vtoroi Vses. Konf. Moscow* 317 (1962); *Chem. Abs.* **62**, 5894 (1965).

16. Borodulina, R. I., Revel'skii, I. A., and Shtylenko, A. D., *Plast. Massy* **49** (1964); *Chem. Abs.* **61**, 11337 (1964).
17. Sakodynskii, K. I., Khokhlova, L. A., Brazhnikov, V. V., and Sevryugova, N. N., *Gazov Khromatogr.* No. 1, 96 (1964); *Chem. Abs.* **67**, 5697 (1967).
18. Nikolaeva, N. M. and Serebryakov, B. R., *Gaz. Khromatogr.* No. 3, 28 (1965); *Chem. Abs.* **66**, 9500 (1967).
19. Nikolaeva, N. M. and Fonkich, A. G., *Gazov Khromatogr.* No. 3, 149 (1965); *Chem. Abs.* **68**, 4451 (1968).
20. Döring, C. E. and Hauthal, H. G., *Acta Chim. Acad. Sci. Hung.* **37**, 125 (1963).
21. van de Craats, F., *Anal. Chim. Acta* **14**, 136 (1956).
22. Zlatkis, A., Chao, G. S., and Kaufman, H. R., *Anal. Chem.* **38**, 2354 (1964).
23. Rotzsche, H., pp. 111–117 in *Gas Chromatography*, edited by M. van Swaay, Butterworths, London (1962).
24. Saha, N. G., Nandi, U. S., and Palit, S. R., *J. Chem. Soc.* **7**, 12 (1958).
25. Bryant, P. J. R., Owen, A. R., and Scanes, F. S., U.S. Patent 3,391, 036 (2/7/68); *Chem. Abs.* **69**, 6427 (1968).
26. Fischer, E., *Z. Chem. Lpz.* **8**, 281 (1968).
27. Schenk, G. H. and Ozolins, M., *Talanta* **8**, 103 (1961).
28. Ozolins, M. and Schenk, G. H., *Anal. Chem.* **33**, 1035 (1961).
29. Schenk, G. H. and Ozolins, M., *Anal. Chem.* **33**, 1562 (1961).
30. Schenk, G. H., Santiago, M., and Wines, P., *Anal. Chem.* **35**, 167 (1963).

PART A

CHEMICAL METHODS

GENERAL INTRODUCTION

ONE may broadly distinguish three types of reaction in the analytical chemistry of any compound class: (1) reactions of the functional group which determines the class (the cyano group in the present case); (2) reactions of parts of the molecule which are influenced (activated) markedly by the proximity of the functional group; (3) reactions of another part or parts of the molecule where the influence of the functional group is scarcely or not discernible.

This third group is theoretically almost limitless but must in practice be reasonably restricted to compounds of some importance (e.g. reactions of the aromatic nucleus in benzonitrile). The demarcation between (2) and (3) is not sharp but the empirical subdivision is useful.

Combinations of two or of all three types occur, especially under more drastic conditions such as in pyrolysis.

The following chapter headings have thus been chosen for discussion of the methods based on:

Reactions of (addition to) the cyano group (Chapter 2).

Reactions of other groups activated or influenced by the cyano group (Chapter 3).

Reactions of other groups in, or parts of, the molecule, sensibly unaffected by the presence of the cyano group (Chapter 4).

Degradation reactions involving the last-named two, during which the cyano group remains intact (Chapter 5).

Combinations of all three types of reaction, resulting in destruction of the cyano group (Chapter 6).

Miscellaneous chemical reactions (Chapter 7).

CHAPTER 2

REACTIONS OF (ADDITION TO) THE CYANO GROUP

Introduction

The cyano group (2.1) is capable of reaction with both nucleophilic and electrophilic reagents:

$$—C{\equiv}N \longleftrightarrow —C^{+}{=}N^{-} \qquad (2.1)$$

Cyano compounds indeed take part in many addition reactions, but most of these are slow and/or incomplete. Those which have been useful for analytical purposes are treated below.

1. Reduction: —CN ⟶ —CH_2—NH_2

Reduction has been utilised in both qualitative and quantitative analysis. Various reducing agents have been used. Table 2.1 summarises some publications and quotes the principle of reduction and the subsequent treatment.

The sodium–alcohol procedure appears to be that principally recommended in handbooks for preparation of derivatives. The nitrile is dissolved in, say, absolute ethanol and freshly cut sodium is added through a reflux condenser. After subsequent acidification, the excess alcohol is distilled off and the amine isolated by rendering alkaline and distilling or extracting.

Clearly there are many other possibilities of detecting or determining the amine formed or of preparing derivatives from it. Any standard procedure is available in principle.

The corresponding secondary amine, or ammonia, may also be formed during reduction (2.2).

$$RC{\equiv}N \longrightarrow RCH_2NH_2 + (RCH)_2NH + NH_3 \qquad (2.2)$$

With sodium–alcohol, sodium cyanide and a hydrocarbon are possible products (2.3).

$$RC{\equiv}N \longrightarrow RH + NaCN \qquad (2.3)$$

TABLE 2.1. ANALYTICAL REDUCTION METHODS FOR NITRILES

Reduction procedure	Analytical aim	Subsequent procedure	Reference
Na–alcohol	Detection of nitriles in distillate heads of light oil	Distilled into dilute HCl and upper layer tested with picric acid	1
HI (sealed tube at 200°)	Quantitative determination	Kjeldahl digestion and determination of N content	2
Na–alcohol	Derivative preparation	Resulting amine, RCH_2NH_2, reacted with C_6H_5NCS, giving thiourea derivative $C_6H_5NH–CS–NHCH_2R$	3
HI(H_2SO_4 + KI, 45 min at *ca.* 100°)	Quantitative determination	"Kjeldahl" digestion and determination of N content	4
$LiAlH_4$	Quantitative determination (some amides and nitriles)	NaOH added and amine distilled into excess H_2SO_4; back-titrated with NaOH to methyl purple	5
$LiAlH_4$ in an ether	Derivative preparation	Amine reacted with 2,4-dinitro-fluorobenzene/acetone, yielding secondary amine product	6
Catalytic hydrogen-ation	Quantitative determination	Amine titrated with $HClO_4$/acetic acid	7
Catalytic hydrogen-ation (finely divided Pd)	Detection (e.g. of benzonitrile) in PC; Pd applied on start line, then hydrogena-ted 30 min	Amine detected through violet yielded with ninhydrin on heating	8
Devarda's alloy	Detection (of benzonitrile)	Benzylamine detected through brown–violet coloration with 1,2-naphthoquinone-4-sulphonate/alkali	9
$TiCl_3$	Detection (of compounds giving amines with $TiCl_3$)	NaOH added, warmed to 70°, and issuing vapours tested with a Ag^+–Mn^{2+}reagent; black Ag^0 and MnO_2 yielded according to: $Mn^{2+} + 2Ag^+ + 4RNH_2 + 2H_2O \rightarrow MnO_2 + 2Ag + 4RNH_3^+$	10
$LiAlH_4$	Quantitative determination	Amine titrated with $HClO_4$–acetic acid	11

These side-reactions could interfere with subsequent stages. Preparation of derivatives in Table 2.1 or any similar preparations (such as amides with acid chlorides or sulphonyl halides) would be susceptible to the first two side-reactions mentioned, since secondary amines and ammonia react likewise; hydrocarbon or sodium cyanide from the third reaction should not interfere. In contrast, the quantitative methods of Table 2.1 are sensibly immune to the first two side-reactions. Titration with acid must give the sum of amines and ammonia; and "Kjeldahl" digestion yields total nitrogen as NH_3. Both results give nitrile equivalents. Formation of hydrocarbon and sodium cyanide means a loss of base, rendering quantitative methods inaccurate; this reduction does not appear to have been used in quantitative work, presumably for this reason. As pointed out by Vanetten and Wiele,[(12)] reduction preceding Kjeldahl digestion is superfluous. The cyano group is converted into ammonia by hydrolysis alone. Prior reduction would be an advantage only with volatile nitriles which would thereby be transformed into amines and retained by the acid.

Lithium aluminium hydride is a special case. It has been suggested and used for determination of active hydrogen as an alternative to the Grignard reagent in the Tschugaev–Zerevitinov procedure. Nitriles containing the —CH—CN group are thus able to react with it in two ways: with reduction of the cyano group and also with the active hydrogen, yielding hydrogen gas. A quantitative method based on consumption of reagent in reduction is consequently possible only with non-enolisable nitriles such as benzonitrile. Publication of such an analytical determination has not been found although sensibly quantitative conversions have been quoted in studies (0·5 mole per cyano group). Thus Zaugg and Horrom[(13)] found mole consumptions of 0·41 0·48 for (2.4),

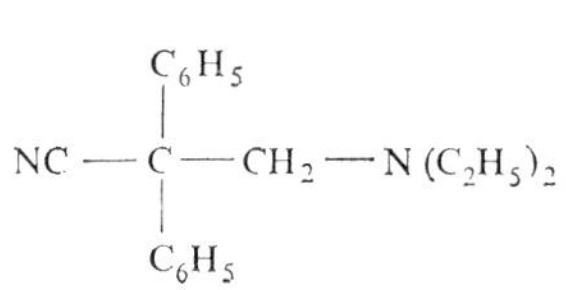

(2.4)

0·29–0·53 for (2.5),

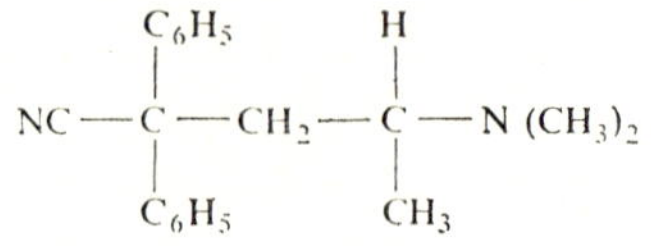

(2.5)

and 0·37–0.45 for (2.6),

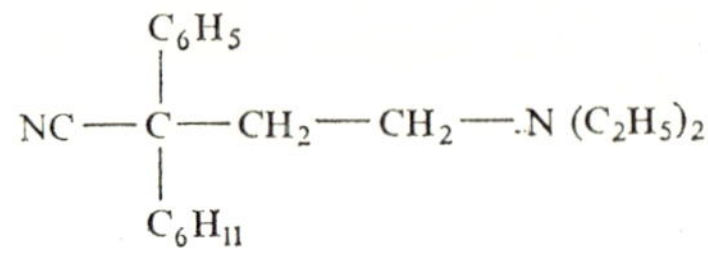

(2.6)

The lower values were under milder conditions such as at room temperature or with reaction for only 1 min at 98°; the higher values were generally obtained with longer reaction times at 98°. Hochstein(14) gives a 0·20–0·28 mole consumption for $(C_6H_5)_3CCN$ at 80–100° in *N*-ethylmorpholine; this is considerably below the theoretical value and may be due to steric hindrance. Even if the approximate values were acceptable, the method based on lithium aluminium hydride consumption suffers, of course, from lack of selectivity; many other groups are likewise reduced. Procedures based on subsequent determination of the amine product are superior, since most of the other reducible groups do not yield amines.

N-cyano compounds, such as cyanamide, have been submitted to reduction as the first stage in analytical procedures but the reaction involves fission of the N–CN link and has been classified in Chapter 5. Feigl and Gentil(15) have thus detected cyanamide through the HCN formed (2.7) and dicyanodiamide through the guanidine yielded; Neubauer(16) determined cyanamide by estimating the ammonia yielded (p. 84).

$$-NH-CN \longrightarrow -NH_2 + HCN\ (\longrightarrow CH_3NH_2) \qquad (2.7)$$

There seems to be no record of quantitative determination of nitriles through the amount of reducing agent consumed, analogous to determinations of nitro, azo, and other compounds with Ti(III), etc.

2. Hydrolysis

$$-C{\equiv}N \longrightarrow -\underset{\underset{O}{\|}}{C}-NH_2 \longrightarrow -COO^- + NH_4^+ \qquad (2.8)$$

Complete conversion into carboxylic acid (or carboxylate) and ammonium ion (or free ammonia) usually requires drastic conditions, such as prolonged heating with 60–70% sulphuric acid or with 40% sodium hydroxide. Attempts have been made to accelerate the overall reaction, e.g. by Travagli[(17)], who found that Hg(II) salts function catalytically. This does not appear to have found any analytical application.

The anion of the acid used for hydrolysis evidently plays an important part. Thus, at high acid concentration, hydrochloric acid is much more effective than sulphuric acid in bringing about hydrolysis. Some of the work on this has been summarised by Kilpatrick.[(18)] Travagli found also that the catalytic effect of Hg(II) salts depended on the nature of the acid and he quoted the sequence $H_2SO_4 > HClO_4 > H_2SeO_4 > H_2CrO_4 > HNO_3 > HCl$ or HBr. One notes that this sequence for sulphuric and hydrochloric acids is the reverse of that found in absence of the mercuric salt catalyst. Detailed investigation of these effects might well yield analytically useful information.

Hydrolysis, first to the amide and then further, has been evaluated analytically in several ways:

(a) Determination of the consumption of a reagent or reagent component, e.g. (i) water, in additions yielding the amide; (ii) alkali, in total hydrolyses yielding the carboxylate anion and ammonia; (iii) acid, in hydrolyses yielding a sufficiently strongly basic product which consumes the acidic reagent.

(b) Detection or determination of a reaction product or its adoption as a derivative, e.g. (i) amide (detected, derivative, determined); (ii) carboxylic acid (derivative, determined); (iii) ammonia (detected, determined).

These procedures are discussed in more detail in the following pages.

(*a*) *Determination of Water Consumed*

Mitchell and Hawkins[(19)] treated nitriles with excess water in a water–acetic acid–boron trifluoride (6·5 ml + 500 ml + 300 g) mixture; after reaction for 2h at 80 ± 2°, pyridine was added to complex the boron trifluoride and thereby prevent esterification of the acetic acid with methanol in the titration reagent subsequently used. The unreacted water was then titrated with Karl Fischer reagent, consisting of iodine–pyridine–methanol–sulphur dioxide. Good results were obtained with 13 nitriles (lower aliphatic nitriles, dinitriles, and some aromatic nitriles). Eberius(20) has used a similar method.

(*b*) *Determination of OH^- Consumed*

The net reaction

$$RCN + H_2O + OH^- \longrightarrow RCOO^- + NH_3 \quad (2.9)$$

can be exploited in several ways (see below), and back-titration of the excess hydroxyl ion is technically the simplest. Ammonia is usually expelled at the higher temperatures used for hydrolysis but should not interfere in back-titration if a suitable indicator is employed or a potentiometric titration is carried out. Concentrated aqueous alkali is used, generally without any solubilising organic solvent. The reaction time required depends on the stability of the nitrile and may be several hours at the boiling-point.

A reaction which may be considered here is due to Radziszewski,(21) who found that nitriles were especially easily converted into amides in alkaline solution at *ca.* 40° in the presence of hydrogen peroxide. The overall change is usually represented by eqn. (2.10).

$$RCN + 2H_2O_2 \longrightarrow RCONH_2 + H_2O + O_2 \quad (2.10)$$

Whitehurst and Johnson(22) adapted this to quantitative analysis. After 5 min reaction at room temperature, they concentrated the reaction solution by heating so as to hydrolyse the amide. Finally they back-titrated with standard sulphuric acid to the phenolphthalein end-point. Good results were obtained with the three lower aliphatic mononitriles and with succinonitrile.

(*c*) *Determination of Acid Consumed*

This method has been described only for dicyanodiamide, where the reaction product, guanylurea (2.11), is comparatively strongly basic and forms a stable salt with acid.

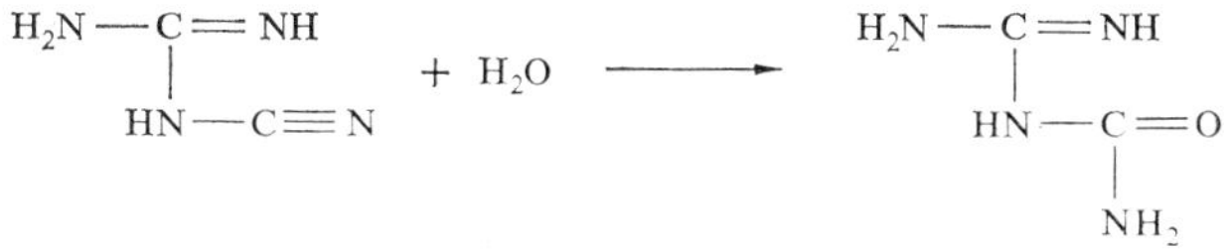

(2.11)

Berlin and Zinov'eva[23] heated for 15 min at 80–85° with 2 N sulphuric or nitric acid, claiming *ca.* 90% hydration. They then back-titrated with calcium or sodium hydroxide to the methyl orange end-point or potentiometrically. Inaba[24] heated with nitric acid for 15 min at 100° in a pressure bottle and back-titrated with alkali.

(*d*) *Amide Formation*

Amides formed under controlled hydration (2.12) conditions can be detected, thus establishing the presence of the nitriles originally. Feigl[25] heats the nitrile with oxalic acid at up to 180°; amides are formed (1.12) which react with the oxalic acid to give oxamide (2.13).

$$RCN + H_2O \longrightarrow RCONH_2 \qquad (2.12)$$

$$2\,RCONH_2 + (COOH)_2 \longrightarrow (CONH_2)_2 + 2\,RCOOH \qquad (2.13)$$

The excess oxalic acid is then removed by sublimation at 200° and the oxamide is detected by the orange colour yielded on heating to 150° with thiobarbituric acid. Feigl was thus able to detect 2–20 μg amounts of some twenty aliphatic nitriles and *N*-cyano compounds. Feigl[26] also quotes a test for cyanoacetic acid which depends likewise on the formation of an intermediate amide. The substance under examination is heated with bromine at 100° until no further free bromine is present. The reaction sequence is presumably as shown in formula (2.13). Some decarboxylation may also occur.

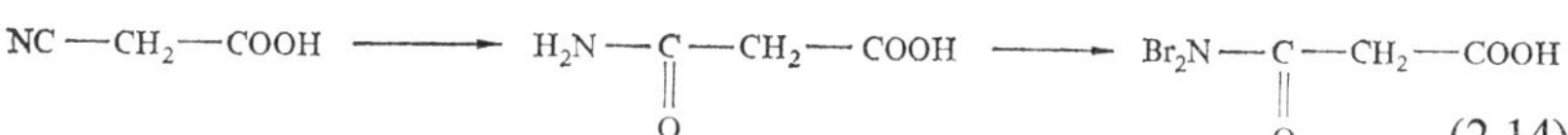

(2.14)

The active bromine attached to nitrogen is then detected by adding starch-iodide; the liberation of iodine yields the well-known blue colour.

Some tests for dicyanodiamide depend on intermediate formation of the corresponding amide, guanylurea (1.11). Thus Bamberger and Seeberger[27] effected hydration by boiling for some hours with dilute acetic acid, then added sodium hydroxide and a little cupric sulphate to yield a pink–red cupric derivative. Grossmann and Schück[28] detected dicyanodiamide through its yellow nickel salt. After adding a few drops of conc. hydrochloric acid, they boiled the solution for 1 min, added a nickel salt and then potassium hydroxide; the nickel derivative then precipitated. A sensitive test described by Feigl and Goldstein[29] depends also on initial hydration to form guanylurea; the detection limit of dicyanodiamide is 25 μg. The hydration is carried out by adding a few drops of hydrochloric acid, then evaporating to dryness. Sodium carbonate and a benzene solution of phenanthraquinone are then added, the solvent is evaporated, and the residue heated to 150°, rising to 190°. A positive test involves the formation of a blue–violet product, yielding a red solution in ether. Feigl and Goldstein make the plausible suggestion that guanidine is first formed through the action of sodium carbonate on the guanylurea and that this then reacts with the quinone to give phenanthraguanidine (2.15).

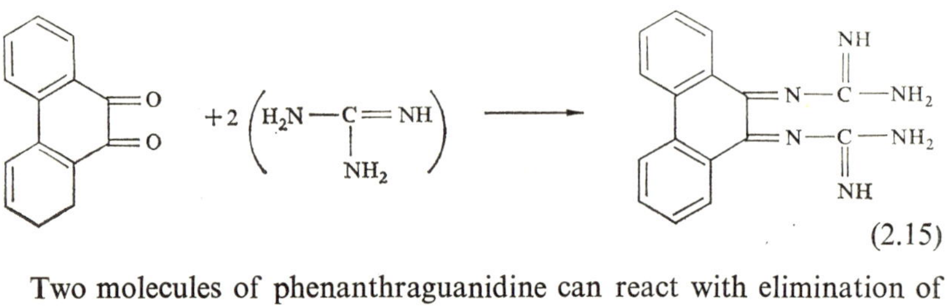

(2.15)

Two molecules of phenanthraguanidine can react with elimination of ammonia between —NH_2 groups, yielding a continuous system of conjugated double bonds which accounts for the intense colour formed.

Amides are excellent derivatives for identification; they are mostly solid and easily crystallised with reasonably high melting points. Both acidic and alkaline hydration conditions can be employed. Verhulst,[30] for example, mixed the amide with conc. sulphuric acid below 25°, then diluted with water, added potassium carbonate, and extracted with an organic solvent. McMaster and Noller[31] used the hydrogen peroxide–alkali reagent.

Dicyanodiamide has also been determined quantitatively by conversion to guanylurea, then estimating this product in one of several ways. A critical stage in this determination is the hydration to the amide, which must be sensibly complete without hydrolysis to acid and ammonia having taken place. Acids are used for this hydration and several sets of conditions have been mentioned already under (c) for quantitative purposes; conditions for detection and derivative preparation have already been given above although quantitative hydration is not necessary for these purposes. Some examples of the determination of dicyanodiamide through its transformation into guanylurea and evaluation of this product are now given:

(*i*) *Gravimetric determination of guanylurea picrate.* Yamazoe and Imai[32] separated the guanylurea from cyanamide by extraction with acetone, converted to guanylurea nitrate with nitric acid, then precipitated the picrate. Buchanan and Barsky[33] treated the sample with 4 N hydrochloric acid at 100° for 15 min to obtain the guanylurea; they neutralised an aliquot of this solution to the phenolphthalein end-point, then added alcoholic picric acid solution, filtering 1 h later.

(*ii*) *Gravimetric determination of nickel derivative.* Garby[34] hydrated with 0·25 N nitric acid; after evaporating to dryness in 2 ± 0·25 h, he added a mannitol–ammonium hydroxide–nickel nitrate reagent, then added sodium hydroxide, slowly precipitating the nickel salt. Watanabe[35] also precipitated the guanylurea as a nickel derivative but determined it by gravimetric estimation of the nickel content as nickel dimethylglyoximate.

(*iii*) *Polarographic determination of N-nitroguanylurea.* Woggon *et al.*[36] have determined dicyanodiamide, used as a stabiliser in plastics and polymers, by treatment with a nitric–sulphuric acid mixture at 50°. This gives *N*-nitro-*N'*-guanylurea (2.16), which was then determined polarographically through reduction of the nitro group.

$$H_2N-\overset{\overset{\displaystyle NH}{\|}}{C}-NH-CO-NH-NO_2 \qquad (2.16)$$

Cyanamide (and its calcium and silver derivatives) has also been quantitatively determined by conversion into the corresponding amide, urea. For this purpose, Fosse *et al.*[37] treated it either with conc. nitric acid for 12 h at room temperature or for 1–2 hr at 40°. They then estimated the urea gravimetrically after its reaction with xanthydrol (2.17) to give dixanthydrylurea.

It is possible that the method of Effront[38] for nitriles depends on initial hydration. He treated the sample with a calcium hypochlorite–sodium

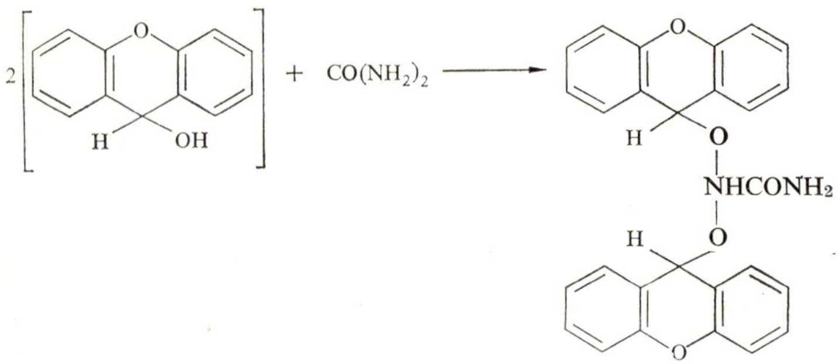

(2.17)

Dixanthydrylurea

hydroxide reagent for 12–15 hr in darkness and determined the excess hypochlorite by adding arsenite and sulphuric acid, back-titrating the excess arsenite with iodine. The reaction sequence is presumably:

$$RCN \rightarrow RCONH_2 \rightarrow RCONHCl + RCONCl_2$$

In the original work it is not clear how far Effront worked with nitriles. They are not mentioned in the title of the article, nor in the examples quoted (only ammonia, hydrazine sulphate and urea), but he makes the general observation that loss of chlorine is directly proportional to the weight of original substance for amines, imines, "nitrile bases", acid amides and amino acids.

(*e*) *Carboxylic Acid Formation*

Carboxylic acids from total hydrolysis of nitriles can serve as derivatives for identification. This is particularly favourable for aromatic nitriles which yield solid acids.

Nitriles may be estimated through determination of the carboxylic acid yielded in quantitative hydrolysis. If acid hydrolysis is used, it will in general be necessary to isolate the carboxylic acid from the reaction mixture containing the mineral acid reagent. The method employed will depend on the nature of the mineral and carboxylic acids. Volatile acids, such as acetic acid from acetonitrile, can be distilled out, preferably after the conc. mineral acid solution has been partly neutralised. Extraction with a suitable solvent, or filtration, may be more suitable with acids of higher molecular weight. Any organic solvent used as a solubiliser during hydrolysis would probably interfere with these separations and should be removed at some earlier stage. As a rule, however, such solvents are not necessary, especially with conc. sulphuric acid.

(f) Ammonia Formation

Evolution of ammonia from a warm alkaline solution is a test for nitriles although it is not wholly specific; acid amides and sulphonamides similarly yield ammonia. Moreover, some nitriles are highly resistant to vigorous treatment, e.g. with 40% alkali. Trofimenko and Sease(39) recommend heating with soda lime as a test for nitriles (and amides). The gaseous products are passed into a cupric sulphate–methanol reagent that yields a blue or purple precipitate. Practically the only interfering compound was ethylenediamine. Eulenhöfer(40) detected dinitriles on thin-layer chromatograms by treating with 2 N H_2SO_4–H_2O_2, drying for 40–60 min in the air and then heating at 120° to yield NH_4^+; this was visualised as a red spot by spraying with a *p*-nitrobenzenediazonium salt and then with alkali.

Separation and estimation of the ammonia formed from complete hydrolysis is probably the most widely used method for the determination of nitriles. Either acid or alkaline conditions can be used. The ammonia has nearly always been determined by classical "Kjeldahl" procedures, i.e. distillation into excess standard acid followed by back-titration with alkali; or distillation into boric acid followed by titration with standard acid. Nessler's reagent has found only occasional use. Some results from the literature are summarised in Table 2.2. These include only nitriles; the *N*-cyano group yields two equivalents of ammonia in reactions which go beyond hydrolysis and this is consequently classified on (p. 93) in Chapter 6.

Siggia and co-workers(55) have developed kinetic methods for analysis of binary mixtures, including mixtures of nitriles or of a nitrile and an amide. The mixture is refluxed in a water–tetrahydrofuran mixture with sodium hydroxide, and the ammonia formed is swept out with a nitrogen current into boric acid at pH 4·00. The pH is maintained at this value by continuous titration with standard hydrochloric acid and the relation of the volume of acid used to the time of reaction is recorded. The hydrolysis of amides and nitriles is a first order process and one can write

$$kt = 2{\cdot}3 \log a/(a - x)$$

where t = time; a = total amide or nitrile; x = amount hydrolysed after time t. a is obtained here by a separate determination of amide + nitrile (e.g. by Kjeldahl procedure) and x is obtained from the acid titration. The plot of log $(a - x)$ against t yields two slopes for binary mixtures of compounds reacting at different rates. Extrapolation of the second slope (the slower reacting compound) to $t = 0$ gives an intercept on the x-axis of log $(a - a_s)$ where a_s is the fraction of the slower-reacting compound. Lower aliphatic nitriles, benzonitrile, and anisonitrile were determined in mixtures, including amides, in this way.

TABLE 2.2. DETERMINATION OF NITRILES THROUGH MEASUREMENT OF AMMONIA EVOLVED IN HYDROLYSIS

Compounds determined	Hydrolysis conditions	Estimation of ammonia	Reference
Nitriles	50% H_2SO_4 in a sealed tube at 150° for 3 hr		41
Benzonitrile in coal tars	Concentrated NaOH		42
Nitriles (also amides)	KOH in benzyl alcohol	Distilled and continuously titrated with H_2SO_4 to methyl orange end-point	43
Trichloroacetonitrile	0·1 N NaOH for 30 min (then distillation for 20 min at *ca.* 100°)	Distilled into boric acid and titrated with standard acid	44
Acrylonitrile in air	50% NaOH, 30% H_2O_2 and some cupric acetate (to prevent polymerisation) added to acid absorption solution; refluxed for 30 min	Distilled into H_2SO_4 and back-titrated	45
Acrylonitrile (treatment with Na-alcohol recommended, to yield less volatile β-ethoxypropionitrile; see Chapter 3, 1(e))	Concentrated H_2SO_4 as in Kjeldahl digestion; also heating with dilute NaOH for less volatile nitriles		46
Saturated nitriles (said to be unsatisfactory for unsaturated)	80% H_2SO_4, as in Kjeldahl procedure		4

TABLE 2.2.–*cont.*

Compounds determined	Hydrolysis conditions	Estimation of ammonia	Reference
Nitriles	90% H_2SO_4 in a sealed tube at 95° for 1–2 hr	Distilled into excess acid and back-titrated	12
Nitriles, e.g. succinodinitrile; (also amides)	Concentrated HCl; 40% NaOH	Distilled into excess acid and back-titrated	47
Nicotinic and isonicotinic acid nitriles	NaOH	Distilled into acid and back-titrated	48
Acrylonitrile in foods, air, and water	Method of ref. 45		49
Acrylonitrile in elastomer polymers	H_2SO_4 + K_2SO_4 + Se + HgO (as Kjeldahl); 6 hr digestion	Distilled into boric acid and titrated	50
Acrylonitrile in copolymers with vinyl-2-picoline	54% H_2SO_4; 2 hr reflux	Distilled into boric acid and titrated	51
Acrylonitrile in copolymers with vinyl-2-picoline	40% NaOH; 4–5 hr	Distilled into acid and back-titrated	52
Benzonitrile	NaOH in an ampoule for 45 min at 140°	Distilled into acid and back-titrated	53
Acetonitrile in trimethylchlorosilane	H_2SO_4 + CrO_3 + $CuSO_4$; 10–20 min	Made alkaline, distilled into standard acid and back-titrated to methyl red–methylene blue end-point	54
Nitrile or nitrile–amide mixtures (kinetic measurements in analysis)	50% KOH in tetrahydrofuran	Continuously distilled into boric acid and titrated with acid to pH 4	55
Adiponitrile in air	NaOH or Na_2CO_3 at *ca.* 100°	Nessler reagent, light absorption at 436 nm	56
Acrylonitrile in air	Concentrated NaOH added to solution in water; 10 min at 100°	Nessler reagent, light absorption at 445 nm	57
Acrylonitrile in air	NaOH, cupric acetate and H_2O_2 added to solution in H_2SO_4	Distilled into excess acid and back-titrated	58
Polyacrylonitrile	H_2SO_4 (Kjeldahl)		59

3. Addition of Hydrogen Sulphide: —CN⟶ —$CSNH_2$

A test for cyanamide, described by Feigl and Gentil,[60] depends on heating with ammonium sulphide, yielding thiourea (2.18).

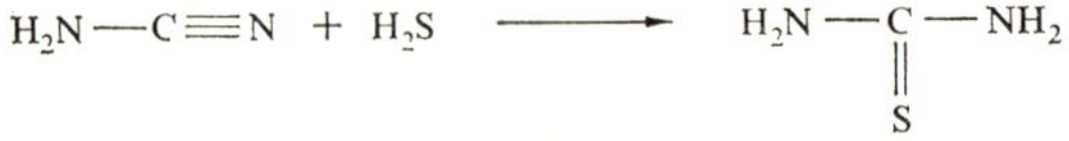

(2.18)

The product is treated with alcoholic monochloroacetic acid solution for 1–2 min at 180°, whereby rhodanine or an oxygen-containing analogue is formed (1.19). This compound, containing an active methylene group, then furnishes a violet colour with 1,2-naphthoquinone-4-sulphonate. The detection limit is 6 μg cyanamide.

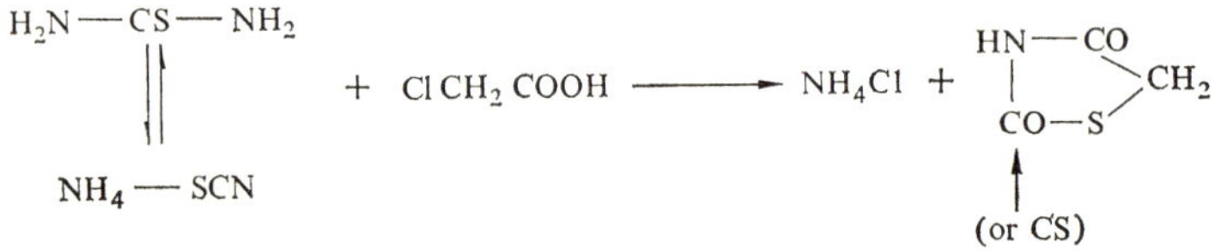

(2.19)

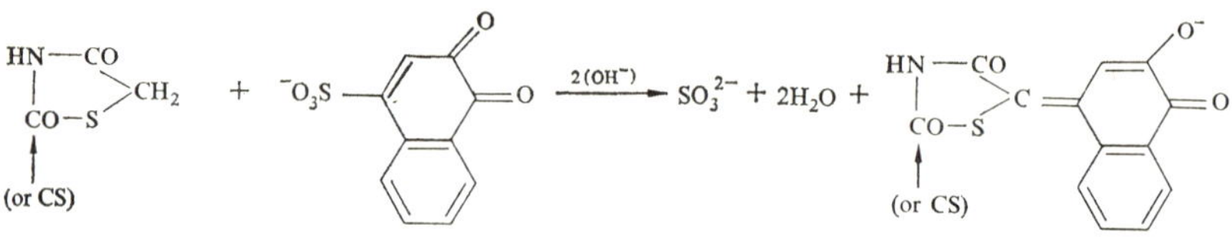

(2.20)

Thioamides have been prepared by Walter and Bode[61] by direct reaction with hydrogen sulphide and also by using diethyl dithiophosphate (1.21) and thioacetamide (1.22).

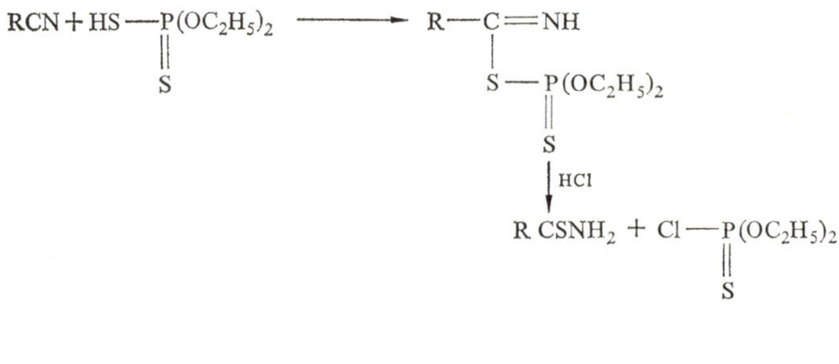

(2.21)

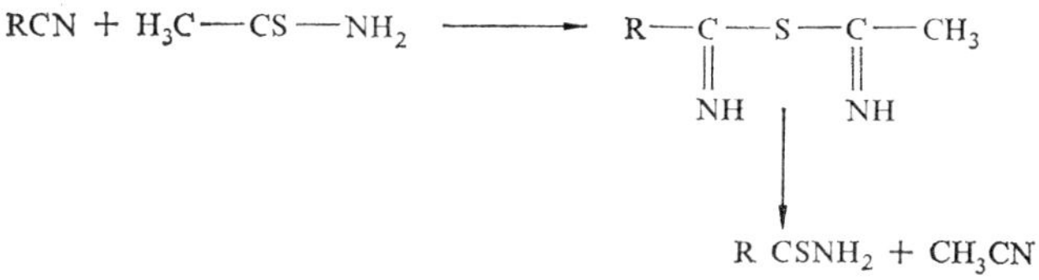

(2.22)

Melting-points were quoted for about twenty-five compounds and the products could serve for identification although this was not in fact proposed by the authors.

4. Addition of Alcohols

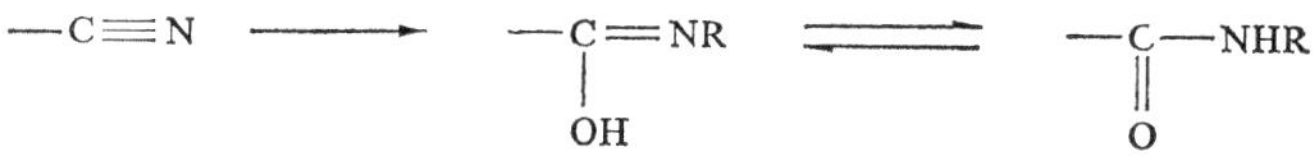

(2.23)

Prajsnar *et al.*[62] have adapted the reaction of Ritter and Minieri[63] for preparation of derivatives of nitriles. They used benzhydrol as reagent, heating with conc. sulphuric acid (2.24) in acetic acid for 30 min at 60° and then leaving for several hours at room temperature before pouring on to ice-water. The precipitate of the *N*-(diphenylmethyl)amides (2.25) was washed and crystallised from alcohol–water.

$$(C_6H_5)_2CHOH + H_2SO_4 \rightleftharpoons (C_6H_5)_2CH{-}OSO_3H + H_2O \qquad (2.24)$$

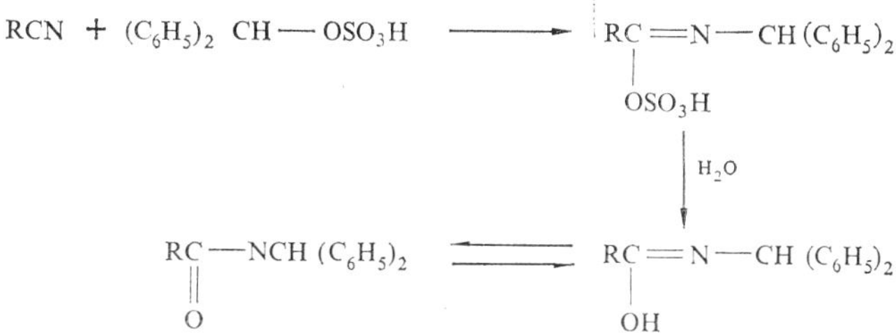

(2.25)

Ritter and Minieri[63] used olefines which presumably reacted with sulphuric acid to yield the sulphate half-esters. Most of their derivatives were liquids or low-melting solids, but high olefines should give more suitable amide products similar to those of Prajsnar and co-workers[62]. A disadvantage is the rather long preparation time.

5. Addition of Ammonia

Although colour reactions for the amidine reaction products are known there seems to be no record of this being adapted to the detection or determination of nitriles by initial treatment with ammonia.

$$NH_2{-}C{\equiv}N + NH_3 \longrightarrow NH_2{-}\underset{\displaystyle NH_2}{\underset{|}{C}}{=}NH \qquad (2.26)$$

A test for cyanamide, based on prior addition of ammonia (2.26) has been described by Feigl *et al.*[64]. The sample is exposed to conc. ammonia for 2–3 min, then left in the air for excess ammonia to disappear. A freshly prepared 5% aqueous solution of sodium 1,2-naphthoquinone-4-sulphonate is then added, yielding a red product (2.27). Cyanamide amounts down to 25 μg can be detected with this procedure; by warming, the sensitivity can be increased to 5 μg amounts. The colour reaction described by Hess[65] is for guanidines and can be employed for detecting any compounds which are convertible into this compound class.

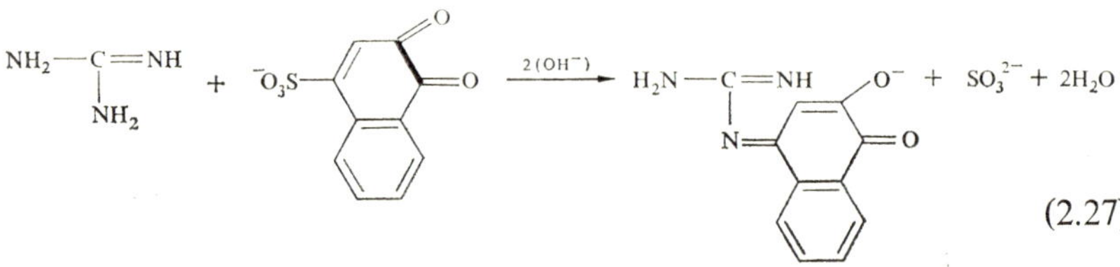

(2.27)

6. Addition of Hydroxylamine

$$-C{\equiv}N \longrightarrow -\underset{\displaystyle NHOH}{\underset{|}{C}}{=}NH \rightleftharpoons -\underset{\displaystyle NOH}{\underset{\|}{C}}{-}NH_2 \qquad (2.28)$$

The products of the reaction of nitriles with hydroxylamine, the amidoximes, yield coloured chelate compounds with various metal cations, notably ferric (2.29).

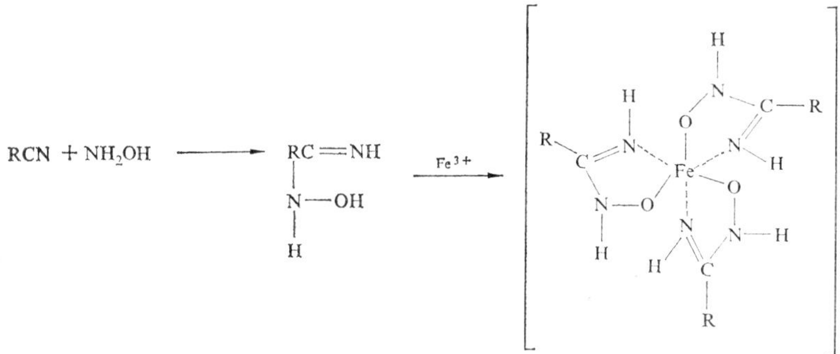

(2.29)

Soloway and Lipschitz[66] investigated this reaction as a test for nitriles. Formation of amidoximes is much slower than that of hydroxamic acids in the first stage of the well-known, analogous test for esters. Soloway and Lipschitz accelerated the reaction rate by using a higher-boiling solvent. Many aliphatic and aromatic nitriles, and also some *N*-cyano compounds such as cyanamide and potassium dicyanoguanidine, gave a positive test (red to violet colour) when hydroxylamine addition was carried out in weakly acid conditions: the sample and 2 ml M hydroxylamine hydrochloride in propylene glycol were mixed with 1 ml M potassium hydroxide solution in the same solvent and boiled for 2–3 min. After cooling, ethanolic ferric chloride was added. (The reaction mixture was not further acidified before adding the ferric chloride because it was found that the ferric chelate was highly sensitive to increased acidity; the final solution is weakly acidic in any case because hydroxylamine hydrochloride is in excess.) Some compounds, such as dicyanodiamide and diethylcyanamide, yielded a positive test only under more acid conditions, when the potassium hydroxide addition was omitted.

Venn[67] has studied this test with a view to quantitative spectrophotometric determination. He confirmed most of the results of Soloway and Lipschitz[66] but was unable to obtain a positive result with acrylonitrile, *m*-nitrobenzonitrile (although the *p*-compound reacted), and diphenylacetonitrile.

Venn first prepared benzamidoxime

$$C_6H_5\text{—}\underset{\displaystyle \text{NHOH}}{\underset{|}{\text{C}}}\text{=NH} \qquad (2.30)$$

and tested its colour production with $Fe^{(3+)}$ in sixteen different solvents. The wavelength of the absorption maximum ranged from *ca.* 400 nm in collidine to *ca.* 620 nm in pyridine, with varying absorptivities. He was able to develop a quantitative method in dimethyl sulphoxide (absorption maximum at 580 nm) and in pyridine, both of which gave relatively stable solutions. The Lambert–Beer relationship was valid using $Fe^{(3+)}$ concentrations between 10^{-5} and 10^{-6} mol/ml and benzamidoxime concentrations up to 3 mg/ml (in dimethyl sulphoxide) or about 0·3 mg/ml (in pyridine). A reaction time of 2 min at 20° was used. The molar absorptivities were about 55 (dimethyl sulphoxide) and 600 (pyridine); the values are thus not high and are less than that of benzhydroxamic acid from benzoate esters (about 200 in dimethyl sulphoxide). Venn prepared and studied other amidoximes, such as succinodiamidoxime, formamidoxime, and acetamidoxime; even less intensive colours were obtained, the molar absorptivities in dimethyl sulphoxide being approximately 35, 20 and 15, respectively.

The conversion of nitrile to amidoxime proved to be the difficult step in the determination. Hydroxylamine reduces $Fe^{(3+)}$ in dimethyl sulphoxide and maxima appear in the visible spectrum which overlap those of the amidoxime–$Fe^{(3+)}$ complex. These interferences did not occur in pyridine solution and Venn therefore tested this medium for benzonitrile. He treated benzonitrile (up to 3 mg) with 100 mg hydroxylamine hydrochloride and 2·131 mg ferric chloride hexahydrate (giving a final concentration of 10^{-6} M $Fe^{(3+)}$), all in a total volume of 3 ml pyridine, and measured the absorbance at 620 nm. He found that reaction was slow and incomplete. Linear calibration curves were indeed obtained but of acceptable sensitivity only after reaction for longer times or higher temperature. Reaction for 3 days at room temperature in darkness or for 2 hr at 100° (the ferric chloride was added after cooling in this case) yielded conversions to benzamidoxime of *ca.* 40% and 20% respectively (based on the benzamidoxime–$Fe^{(3+)}$ curves). Amounts of *ca.* 0·1–1 mg/ml benzonitrile could be determined in this empirical procedure. Longer reaction times, especially at higher temperature, would probably endanger reproducibility through losses of nitrile and or amidoxime. Propionitrile similarly yielded a linear calibration curve after reaction for several days at room temperature, but attempts to accelerate the reaction at increased temperature led to decomposition of the coloured complex.

Robertson *et al.*[(68)] have recently published a method for amides, amino acids, and acetonitrile, based on measurement of the light absorbance of ferric derivatives of acetamidoxime. They mixed their sample (in aqueous solution) with 4 M hydroxylamine hydrochloride and 8 M sodium hydroxide (2 ml of each solution). This was heated for 16 min at 98° in a closed vessel, then 2 ml of 8 M hydrochloric acid and 2 ml of a 0·74 M ferric chloride solution in 0·1 M hydrochloric acid (pH 1·03–1·07) were added. After 30 sec, the absorbance was measured at 530 nm. Venn found that the acetamidoxime–$Fe^{(3+)}$ complex had an absorption maximum at 470 nm in methanol; his results for benzamidoxime and formamidoxime showed that the absorption maxima in water are 30–40 nm lower than in methanol; one would thus expect acetamidoxime to have an absorption maximum at 430–440 nm, 100 nm lower than the wavelength chosen by Robertson *et al.* Venn found that a decrease in pH caused a bathochromic displacement of the absorption maximum to higher wavelengths; the final solution of Robertson *et al.* is probably appreciably more acid and this may explain the discrepancy. It is, however, interesting that Venn also found that even traces of mineral acids, such as hydrochloric acid, destroyed the coloured complex, and, further, that addition of neutral salts suppressed colour formation; the solution from the acetonitrile determination must contain a high concentration of sodium chloride, and it is thus surprising that acetonitrile concentrations down to 0·008 M could be determined.

A standard method for the determination of carbonyl compounds is based on determination of the acid liberated in reaction (2.31).

$$>C{=}O + H_2NOH.HX \longrightarrow >C{=}NOH + H_2O + HX \qquad (2.31)$$

Venn has carried out some orientation experiments on the adaptation of this principle to the determination of benzonitrile. He used a 3×10^{-3} M solution of hydroxylamine hydrochloride in pyridine and in dimethyl sulphoxide and measured the absorbance of various indicators as a function of the hydrochloric acid liberated. *o*-Phenylenediamine proved to be the best indicator. Slow and incomplete reaction created the same problem as above in the colorimetric method but an empirical procedure should be possible, based on the increased absorbance of the indicator. Much remains to be investigated in connection with amidoxime formation but unless the reaction can be appreciably accelerated, the prospects of developing a suitable method are not rosy.

7. Addition of Hydrazine

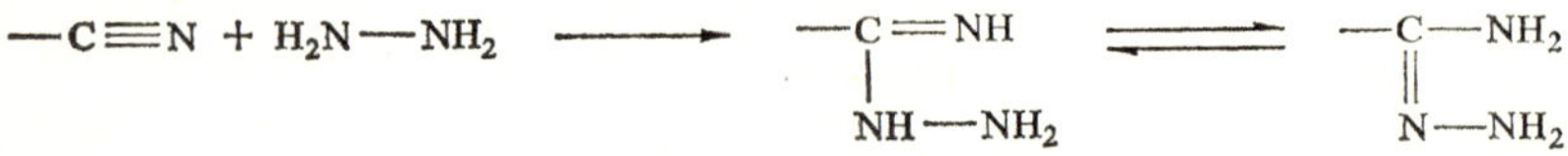

(2.32)

The reaction products, amidrazones, form coloured complexes with $Fe^{(3+)}$. Thus Venn[67] observed an absorption maximum at 510 nm after adding ferric chloride to a heated mixture of benzonitrile and hydrazine hydrate in water. Numerous side-reactions may occur, such as those leading to various triazole derivatives, so that a colorimetric method probably cannot be worked out. It is of interest that when hydrazine is replaced by phenylhydrazine, no colour difference is observed between sample and blank on adding ferric ion; the phenyl group presumably hinders complex formation.

8. Addition of Mercaptans

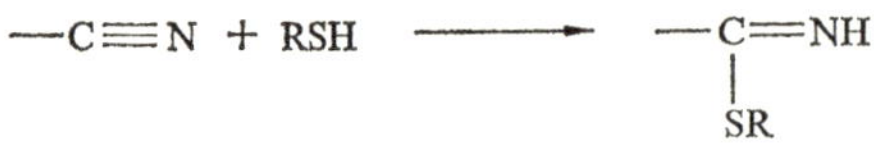

(2.33)

Condo and co-workers[69] have used mercaptoacetic acid to prepare derivatives (2.34) from nitriles (9 aliphatic and 4 aromatic). The reaction was carried out in dry diethyl ether, saturated with hydrogen chloride. Crystals separated on standing in an ice-water bath.

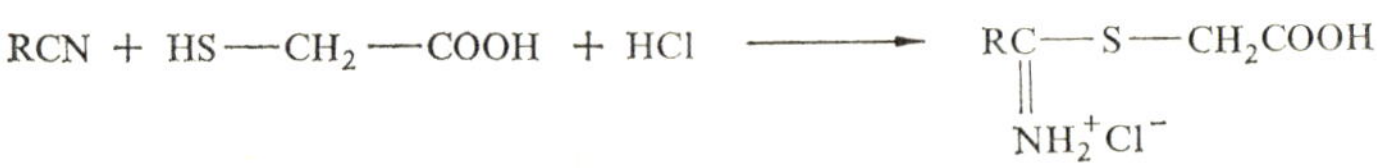

(2.34)

Decomposition-points rather than melting-points were determined, and equivalent weights were estimated by titration with sodium hydroxide.

9. Addition of Polyphenols

Polyphenols react with nitriles in the presence of zinc chloride and hydrogen chloride to yield ketimines (Houben–Hoesch reaction); the ketimines may be converted into ketones by hydrolysis (2.35).

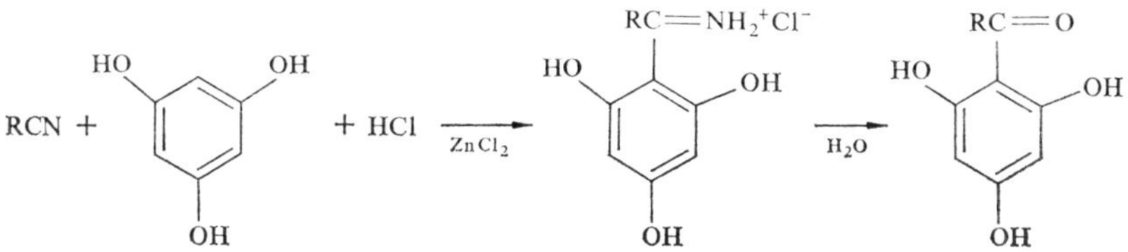

(2.35)

Howells and Little[70] used phloroglucinol, dissolving it and the nitrile in ether, adding zinc chloride and passing in hydrogen chloride, all under anhydrous conditions. The ketimines separated as oils and were dissolved in water and heated. Crystalline ketone derivatives were obtained in 30–90% yield. Only six nitriles were investigated (aceto-, propio-, n-butyro-, n-valero-, n-capro- and i-capronitriles) so that limited comparison data are available for identification.

10. Addition of Grignard Reagent

Shriner and Turner[71] proposed the addition of a Grignard reagent to the nitrile group as the first stage in the identification of nitriles. They used phenyl magnesium bromide and hydrolysed the product to a phenyl ketone (yields of 50–90%) (2.36).

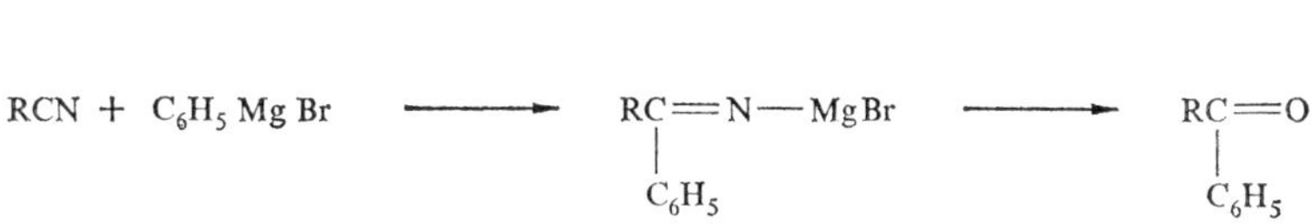

(2.36)

The ketones may be converted into solid derivatives such as semicarbazones, if necessary. The same six nitriles as under section 9 above were investigated so that only restricted data are available here too.

Soltys[72] adapted the active hydrogen determination of Tschugaev and Zerewitinov to the quantitative evaluation of functional groups, including the cyano group, which add on the Grignard reagent. The principle of his method was the use of excess reagent for an adequate reaction time, followed by determination of the unused reagent by adding a compound containing active hydrogen (water, an alcohol or amine such as aniline) and measuring the methane evolved:

$$R---H + CH_3MgI \longrightarrow CH_4 + R---MgI \qquad (2.37)$$

The difference from the amount of methane yielded by an identical aliquot of original Grignard reagent represents the amount consumed in the addition reaction.

Subsequent workers have studied this adaptation but its application to cyano compounds has been scanty. Macinnity and Cloke[73] devised a modified apparatus and quote γ-chlorobutyronitrile among their examples of determination (0·97 ± 0·02 moles added). Zaugg and Horrom[13] compared in detail the use of methyl magnesium iodide and lithium aluminium hydride for determination of active hydrogen and of functional groups which add on or are reduced. Amongst several examples of other compound classes, they cite two nitriles which react fairly completely: compound (2.4) reacts with 1·01 mole in 1 hr at 98°, although with only 0·49 mole in 20 min at room temperature; and (2.5) reacts with 0·97 mole in 1 hr at 98° and 0·64 mole in 5 min at that temperature. The nitrile (2.6) is evidently sterically hindered; after 5 min at 98°, only 0·04 mole had reacted and, even after 30 min, only 0·05 mole.

Nitriles having α-hydrogen atoms may react in two ways to give (i) addition to the cyano group and (ii) methane formation if the hydrogen is sufficiently activated. All nitriles contain this structure except those containing a cyano group directly attached to an aromatic or heterocyclic nucleus or a few comparatively rarely encountered tertiary types such as those just mentioned. This complicates the application of the method. Thus Zaugg and Horrom[13] found, for example, that diphenylacetonitrile in 20 min at room temperature reacted to the extent of 59% to yield methane and 39% in addition; phenyl cyclohexylacetonitrile showed the corresponding values of 12% and 63% in 5 min at 98°. Quantitative application of this principle thus has its limitations.

11. Preparation of N-(2-Chloroalkyl) amides

Cairns *et al.*[74] have prepared *N*-(2-chloroalkyl) amides from nitriles by reaction with olefines–halogen. The three-component ionic reaction (2.38) probably takes place.

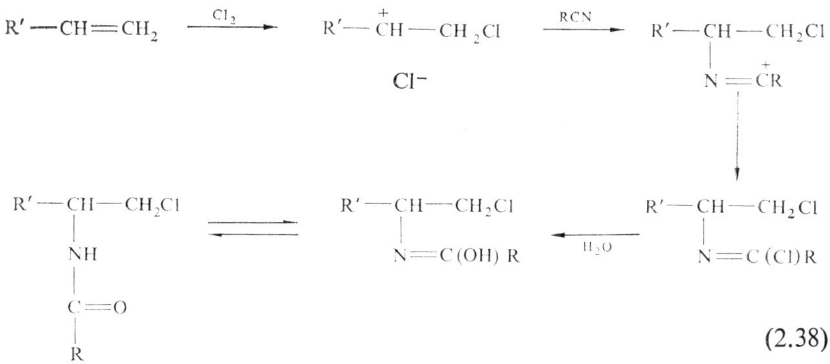

(2.38)

Cairns *et al.* quoted the melting-points of a number of derivatives and, although they did not suggest any analytical application, this would appear to be a practical possibility.

12. Formation of Metal Complexes

Hartung and Jewell[75] made use of complexes of nitriles (and some other nitrogen-containing compounds) to separate them from the hydrocarbons in petroleum products such as hydrogenated furnace oil. The products were first washed with hydrochloric acid to remove bases and were then treated with ferric and/or zinc chloride. Nitriles (also indoles, carbazoles, and phenazines) yielded solid complexes which were dried at 80° and were ultimately decomposed by heating at 450° in nitrogen; tests with benzonitrile, naphthonitriles and other aromatic nitriles showed that recovery was without structural change. The indoles, carbazoles and phenazines were then separated from the condensate with 72% perchloric acid and the residual nitriles were separated by fractional elution through alumina or by gas chromatography. Final identification was with the help of ultraviolet or mass spectra.

Other complexing agents such as chlorides of cobalt, copper, and mercury, and also heteropoly acids, were much less effective than the ferric and zinc halides.

The reaction (2.39) may be classified as one of addition.

$$R{-}C{\equiv}N \xrightarrow{FeCl_3} Ar{-}C{\equiv}N^{+}{-}FeCl_2 \qquad (2.39)$$

$$\longleftrightarrow Ar{-}\overset{+}{C}{=}N{-}FeCl_2 \longleftrightarrow Ar^{+}{=}C{=}N{-}FeCl_2 \quad [Cl^{-}]$$

References

1. Desvergnes, L., *Ann. Chim. Anal. Chim. Appl.* **4**, (2) 129 (1925).
2. Friedrich, A., Kühaas, E., and Schürch, R., *Z. Physiol. Chem.* **216**, 68 (1933).
3. Cutter, H. B. and Taras, M., *Ind. Eng. Chem., Anal. Ed.* **13**, 830 (1941).
4. Rose, E. L. and Ziliotto, H., *Ind. Eng. Chem., Anal. Ed.* **17**, 211 (1945).
5. Siggia, S. and Stahl, C. R., *Anal. Chem.* **27**, 550 (1955).
6. Bräuniger, H. and Spangenberg, K., *Pharmazie* **12**, 488 (1957).
7. Meyers, R. T., *Ohio J. Sci.* **58**, 34 (1958).
8. Kaufmann, H. P. and Chowdbury, D. K., *Chem. Ber.* **91**, 2117 (1958).
9. Feigl, F., *Anal. Chem.* **33**, 1118 (1961).
10. Pesez, M., Bartos, J., and Lampetaz, J.-C., *Bull. Soc. Chim. France* 719 (1962).
11. Huber, W., *Z. Anal. Chem.* **197**, 236 (1963).
12. Vanetten, C. H. and Wiele, M. B., *Anal. Chem.* **23**, 1338 (1951).
13. Zaugg, H. E. and Horrom, B. W., *Anal. Chem.* **20**, 1026 (1948).
14. Hochstein, F. A., *J. Am. Chem. Soc.* **71**, 305 (1949).
15. Feigl, F. and Gentil, V., *Mikrochim. Acta* 44 (1959).
16. Neubauer, H., *Z. Angew. Chem.* **33**, 247 (1920).
17. Travagli, G., *Gazz. Chim. Ital.* **66**, 525 (1936); *Ann. Univ. Studi Ferrara* **6**, (1947); *Ann. Univ. Studi Ferrara* **8**, pt. 1 (1949–50); *Atti Accad. Sci. Ferrara* 27 (1949–50); *Gazz. Chim. Ital.* **87**, 673 (1957).
18. Kilpatrick, M. L., *J. Am. Chem. Soc.* **69**, 42 (1947).
19. Mitchell, J. and Hawkins, W., *J. Am. Chem. Soc.* **67**, 777 (1945).
20. Eberius, E., *Chem. Tech.* (*Berlin*) **4**, 291 (1952).
21. Radziszewski, B., *Chem. Ber.* **18**, 355 (1885).
22. Whitehurst, D. H. and Johnson, J. B., *Anal. Chem.* **30**, 1332 (1958).
23. Berlin, A. A. and Zinov'eva, Z. A., *Zh. Obshch. Khim.* **17**, 43 (1947).
24. Inaba, H., *Japan Analyst* **3**, 111 and 195 (1954); *Chem. Abs.* **48**, 9866 (1954) and **49**, 4458 (1955).
25. Feigl, F. and Amaral, J. R., "*Spot Tests in Organic Analysis*", 7th English Edition, Elsevier Pub. Co. (1966), p. 264.
26. Feigl, F. and Del'Acqua, A., *ibid.*, p. 551.
27. Bamberger, E. and Seeberger, S., *Chem. Ber.* **26**, 1583 (1893).
28. Grossmann, H. and Schück, B., *Chem. Ber.* **39**, 3357 (1906).
29. Feigl, F. and Goldstein, D., *Z. Anal. Chem.* **178**, 265 (1961).
30. Verhulst, J., *Bull. Soc. Chim. Belge* **39**, 563 (1930); **40**, 475 (1931).
31. McMaster, L. and Noller, C. R., *J. Indian Chem. Soc.* **12**, 652 (1935).
32. Yamazoe, F. and Imai, J., *Bunseki Kagaku* (*Japan Analyst*) **9**, 877 (1960).

33. BUCHANAN, G. H. and BARSKY, G., *J. Am. Chem. Soc.* **52**, 198 (1930).
34. GARBY, C. D., *Ind. Eng. Chem.* **17**, 266 (1925).
35. WATANABE, S., *J. Taihoku Soc. Agr. Forestry* **1**, 171 (1936); *Chem. Abs.* **31**, 69 (1937).
36. WOGGON, H., KOEHLER, U., and KORN, O., *Ernährungsforschung* **11**, 548 (1966).
37. FOSSE, R., HAGÈNE, P., and DUBOIS, R., *Comptes Rendus* **179**, 214, 408 (1924).
38. EFFRONT, J., *Chem. Ber.* **37**, 4290 (1904).
39. TROFIMENKO, S. and SEASE, J. W., *Anal. Chem.* **30**, 1432 (1958).
40. EULENHÖFER, H. G., *J. Chromatog.* **36**, 198 (1968).
41. GUILLEMAND, H., *Bull. Soc. Chim.* (4) **1**, 196 (1907).
42. GOL'DIN, G., *Zh. Obshch. Khim.* **8**, 557 (1935).
43. PALFRAY, L., SABETAY, S., and ROVIRA, S., *Comptes Rendus* **209**, 754 (1939).
44. LUBATTI, O. F. and HARRISON, A., *J. Soc. Chem. Ind., London* **63**, 140 (1944).
45. PETERSEN, G. W. and RADKE, H. H., *Ind. Eng. Chem., Anal. Ed.* **16**, 63 (1944).
46. DAVIS, H. S. and WIEDEMANN, O. F., *Ind. Eng. Chem.* **37**, 482 (1945).
47. ANDRADE, J. L. *et al.*, *Rev. Sanidad y Asistencia Social (Venezuela)* **21**, 231 (1956).
48. CZERWINSKI, W., *Chem. Anal. (Warsaw)* **3**, 53 (1958).
49. JEDLICKA, V., PASEK, V., and GOLA, J., *J. Hyg. Epidemiol. Microbiol. Immunol.* **2**, 116 (1958); *Chem. Abs.* **52**, 17545 (1958).
50. BURLEIGH, J. E., MCKINNEY, O. F., and BARKER, M. G., *Anal. Chem.* **31**, 1684 (1959).
51. STAFFORD, C. and TOREN, P. E., *Anal. Chem.* **31**, 1687 (1959).
52. EMELIN, E. A., SVISTUNOVA, G. and TSARFIN, YA. A., *Zavod. Lab.* **27**, 283 (1961).
53. GORELOV, P. N., *Zavod. Lab.* **28**, 668 (1962).
54. SYAVTSILLO, S. V., LUSKINA, B. M., and KARABASHKINA, L. N., *Plast. Massy.* No. 2, 24 (1962).
55. SIGGIA, S., HANNA, J. G., and SERENCHA, N. M., *Anal. Chem.* **36**, 227 (1964).
56. BELYAKOV, A. A., *Tr. Po. Khim. i Khim. Tekhnol.* 139 (1964); *Chem. Abs.* **62**, 2170, (1965).
57. ROGACZEWSKA, T., *Med. Pracy* **16**, 465 (1965).
58. THIEDE, H. and FRANZEN, E., *Wiss. Z. Martin-Luther Univ., Halle-Wittenberg, Math.-Nat. Reihe* **14**, 177 (1965).
59. DANKE, M., *Faserforsch. Textilchemie* **18**, 123 (1967).
60. FEIGL, F. and GENTIL, V., *Anal. Chem.* **29**, 1715 (1957).
61. WALTER, W. and BODE. K.-D., *Z. Angew. Chem.* **78**, 517 (1966).
62. PRAJSNAR, B., MASLANKIEWICZ, A., and NAJZAREK, Z., *Chem. Anal. (Warsaw)* **10**, 1221 (1965).
63. RITTER, J. J. and MINIERI, P. P., *J. Am. Chem. Soc.* **70**, 4045 (1948).
64. FEIGL, F., GOLDSTEIN, D., and LIBERGOTT, E., *Chemist-Analyst* **53**, 37 (1964).
65. HESS, W. C., *Proc. Soc. Exptl. Biol. Med.* **33**, 106 (1935).
66. SOLOWAY, S. and LIPSCHITZ, A., *Anal. Chem.* **24**, 898 (1952).
67. VENN, I., *Diplomarbeit*, University of the Saar, Saarbrücken (1968).
68. ROBERTSON, E. B., SYKES, B. D., and DUNFORD, H. B., *Anal. Biochem.* **9**, 158 (1964).
69. CONDO, F. E., HINKEL, E. T., FASSERO, A. and SHRINER, R. L., *J. Am. Chem.* **59**, 230 (1937).
70. HOWELLS, H. P. and LITTLE, J. G., *J. Am. Chem. Soc.* **54**, 2451 (1932).
71. SHRINER, R. L. and TURNER, T. A., *J. Am. Chem. Soc.* **52**, 1267 (1930).
72. SOLTYS, A., *Mikrochemie* **20**, 107 (1936).
73. MACINNITY, P. M. and CLOKE, J. B., *Anal. Chem.* **20**, 978 (1948).
74. CAIRNS, T. L., GRAHAM, P. J., BARRICK, P. L. and SCHREIBER, R. S., *J. Org. Chem.* **17**, 751 (1952).
75. HARTUNG, G. K. and JEWELL, D. M., *Anal. Chim. Acta* **27**, 219 (1962).

CHAPTER 3

REACTIONS OF GROUPS ACTIVATED BY THE CYANO GROUP

Introduction

Three groups are considered here: the olefinic —C═C— group in the so-called α,β-unsaturated nitriles; the activated methylene or methine group in compounds possessing the structural unit $—CH_2—CN$ or ═CH—CN; and the amino or imino group directly linked to a cyano group, $H_2N—CN$ or —NH—CN.

1. α, β-Unsaturated Nitriles

Nucleophilic reagents such as amines, hydroxylamine, bisulphite, and mercaptans add on readily to the —C═C— group, activated by —CO—, $—NO_2$, —CN groups, etc. Most work has been done on the more frequently encountered α, β-unsaturated carboxylic acids, esters, and carbonyl compounds. The nitriles have, however, not been wholly neglected and some publications are summarised in the sections below. Most of these articles have concerned quantitative determinations and one feels that more use might be made of the reactions for purposes of identification.

Polarographic reduction of α,β-unsaturated nitriles, one of the most useful methods for their determination, is dealt with in Chapter 11.

Acrylonitrile is the outstanding example of this type of nitrile and practically all the analytical work has concerned it.

(a) *Addition of Amines*

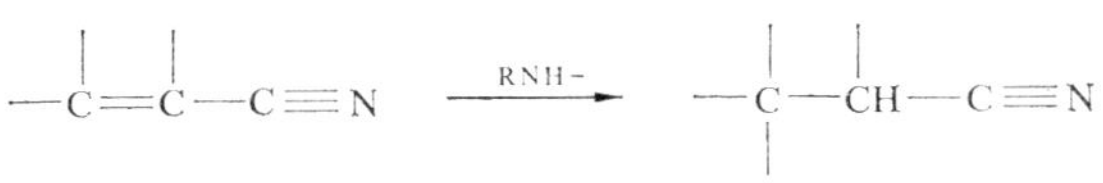

(3.1)

Brockway[1] detected and identified acrylonitrile, even in 1% solutions, by adding piperidine and then, after some minutes, excess 10–12% aqueous picric acid solution. The precipitate of the picrate of β-piperidinopropionitrile was crystallised from ethanol and melts at 161–162°. The only other example tested was methacrylonitrile which yields a picrate precipitate (m.p. 140–141°) only after several days' reaction time with the amine.

Brockway used morpholine also, the corresponding picrate of β-morpholinopropionitrile melting at 138–140°. Methiodides and hydrochlorides were also prepared from both acrylonitrile derivatives, but the picrates are the easiest to prepare.

In quantitative procedures, secondary amines such as morpholine have usually been employed; glycine was used in one method. Two standard procedures have been used: acetylation of the unused amine by adding acetic anhydride and then titrating the tertiary amine product with standard acid; or determination of the unreacted amine reagent. Table 3.1 contains some abstracted publications.

TABLE 3.1. DETERMINATION OF NITRILES BY ADDITION OF AMINES

Nitrile	Reagent	Conditions	Final stage	Reference
Acrylonitrile	Glycine	+ KOH; 1hr at room temperature	Excess glycine determined by measuring N_2 liberated with HNO_2 (Van Slyke)	2
Acrylonitrile, methacrylonitrile, allyl cyanide (which isomerises under the conditions used)	Morpholine	In acetic acid as solvent and catalyst; from 5 min at 25° to to 4 hr at 98°	Acetylated with acetic anhydride in acetonitrile and titrated with HCl–methanol to methyl orange–Xylene Cyanol or conductometrically	3
Acrylonitrile	Piperidine	In dioxan, + acetic acid as catalyst; 30 min	Acetylated and titrated with HCl–methanol to methyl red–methylene blue	4
Acrylonitrile	Hexamethyleneimine	In anhydrous methanol; 4 hr	Acetylated and titrated with HCl–methanol to methyl red–methylene blue	5

TABLE 3.1—*cont.*

Nitrile	Reagent	Conditions	Final stage	Reference
Acrylonitrile (sub-micro)	Morpholine	In methylcellosolve + some acid; 30–90 min	Titrated with $HClO_4$ to thymol blue	6
Tetracyanoethylene; 1-aminophenol-2,2-dicyanoethylene	Morpholine	In diethylene glycol dimethyl ether; 30 min	Titrated with $HClO_4$ to thymol blue	6

(*b*) *Addition of Hydroxylamine*

$$-\overset{|}{C}=\overset{|}{C}-C\equiv N + NH_2OH \longrightarrow -\underset{\underset{NHOH}{|}}{\overset{|}{C}}-\overset{|}{C}H-CN \qquad (3.2)$$

Terent'ev *et al.*[7] have developed a method for quantitative determination of acrylonitrile which is based on this reaction. They used excess hydroxylamine in dioxan solution in the presence of alkali catalyst. After the rather long reaction time of 12 hr, acetone was added to remove excess hydroxylamine and the mixture was titrated potentiometrically with standard hydrochloric acid. Two potential jumps were obtained, corresponding to consumption of excess alkali and then to reaction of the basic derivative.

(*c*) *Addition of Bisulphite*

$$-\overset{|}{C}=\overset{|}{C}-C\equiv N \xrightarrow{HSO_3^-} -\underset{\underset{SO_3^-}{|}}{\overset{|}{C}}-\overset{|}{C}H-CN \qquad (3.3)$$

Several quantitative methods have been published which depend on the formation of a bisulphite compound. Mostly sulphite has been used, the formation of the bisulphite compound (3.4) being then accompanied by decrease in acidity:

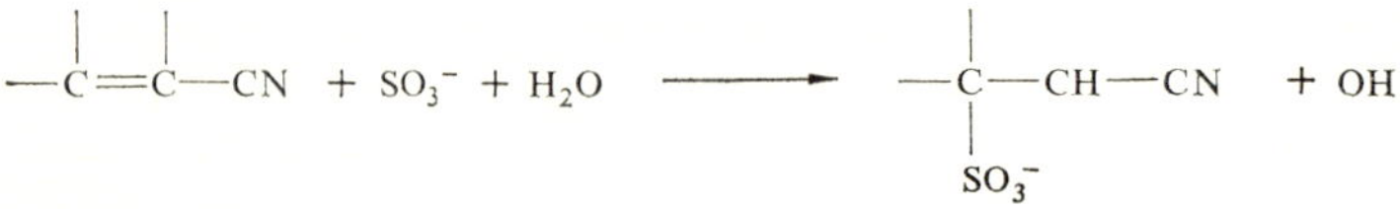

(3.4)

This is similar to procedures for the determination of carbonyl compounds and similar conclusions are possible, namely: measurement of unused bisulphite; determination of $OH^{(-)}$ formed; determination of residual acid when the starting solution contains excess standard acid. Examples are given in Table 3.2.

TABLE 3.2. DETERMINATION OF NITRILES* BY ADDITION OF BISULPHITE

Reaction conditions	Final stage	Reference
Aqueous solution, + $SO_3^{(2-)}$ + excess H_2SO_4; 5–30 min at 25°	Titrated unused acid with alkali to Alizarin Yellow R–Xylene Cyanol end-point	8
In dioxan, + $SO_3^{(2-)}$; 60–90 min	Titrated with HCl to thymolphthalein end-point	9
In dioxan, + $SO_3^{(2-)}$; 60–90 min	Titrated with H_2SO_4 to thymolphthalein–Alizarin Yellow R end-point	10
Aqueous solution + standard $NaHSO_3$ +15 min at *ca.* 100°	Unused bisulphite titrated with alkali to thymolphthalein end-point	11
In dioxan, + $SO_3^{(2-)}$; 5 min at room temperature	Aliquot diluted with water and titrated potentiometrically with HCl	12
As in ref. 10 (determination of residual acrylonitrile from estimation of alcohols through reaction with excess nitrile–KOH)	Titrated with HCl to thymolphthalein–Alizarin Yellow R end-point	13
Aqueous solution, + $SO_3^{(2-)}$ + excess H_2SO_4; 10 min at 25°	Titrated unused acid with NaOH to thymolphthalein or Alizarin Yellow R end-point	14
Sample, + $SO_3^{(2-)}$ + excess H_2SO_4; 1 hr	Titrated unused acid with NaOH to Alizarin Yellow end-point	15

* Acrylonitrile in all instances except in the last which was a determination of α-(dimethoxymethyl)acrylonitrile (3.5) in a study of mixtures with α-(dimethoxymethyl)-

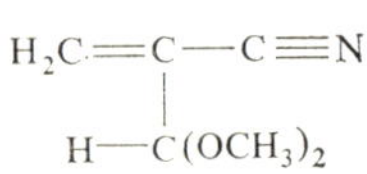

(3.5)

β-propionitrile and *cis*- and *trans*-α-(methoxymethyl)-β-propionitriles.

Systematic work remains to be done on other unsaturated nitriles, which, apart from the last example in Table 3.2, do not appear to have been investigated.

(*d*) *Addition of Mercaptans*

$$-\overset{|}{C}=\overset{|}{C}-CN + RSH \longrightarrow -\underset{SR}{\overset{|}{\underset{|}{C}}}-\underset{H}{\overset{|}{\underset{|}{C}}}-CN \qquad (3.6)$$

This reaction has been used more than any other for the determination of α,β-unsaturated nitriles (and other α,β-unsaturated compounds such as ketones and esters). A basic catalyst is necessary. The chief sources of error are atmospheric oxidation of the mercaptan and the addition of other molecules, notably of alcohol solvent molecules, to the double bond. Short reaction times minimise the danger of oxidation. The cyano-alkylation error can be suppressed by preventing nitrile and alcohol solvent from coming into contact in the presence of basic catalyst and in the absence of mercaptan; the mercaptan should always be present before the addition of catalyst.

As seen from tabulated results below (Table 3.3) dodecyl mercaptan and mercaptoacetate are the two reagents which have been used. The measurement stage has been evaluation of the unreacted mercaptan, for which standard methods have been used. As in procedures (*a*) to (*c*), practically all determinations reported have involved acrylonitrile.

Štěpánek and co-workers[24, 25] have detected traces of acrylonitrile by boiling with thiourea/hydrochloric acid in ethanol or isopropanol for 30 min, yielding 2-(2-cyanoethyl)isothiouronium chloride (3.7).

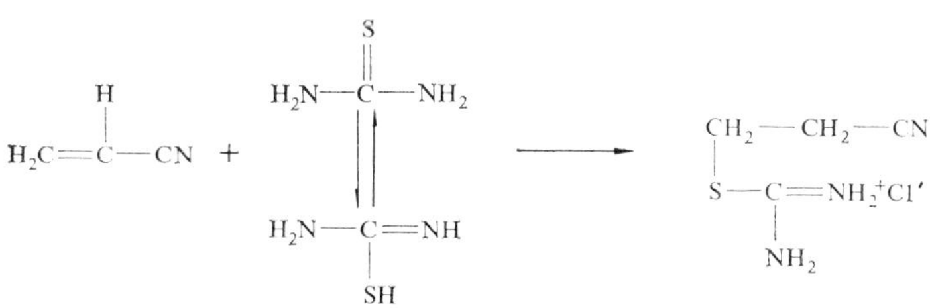

(3.7)

This product was separated by descending paper chromatography using

TABLE 3.3. DETERMINATION OF NITRILES BY ADDITION OF MERCAPTANS

Nitrile	Reagent	Reaction conditions	Determination of unused reagent	Reference
Acrylonitrile	Dodecyl mercaptan	Sample + reagent in ethanol or isopropanol, then + basic catalyst (KOH or trimethyl benzyl ammonium hydroxide); 2 min reaction time using *ca.* 2 × theoretical amount of mercaptan	+ Acetic acid and titrated with iodine (for 20–200 mg amounts); + acetic acid + NH_4OH and titrated amperometrically with $AgNO_3$ (for 2–30 mg amounts)	16
Acrylonitrile; 1-cyano-1,3-butadiene	Dodecyl mercaptan	In dioxan or isopropanol, + KOH–isopropanol; 2 min	+ HCl + isopropanol and titrated with bromate	17
Acrylonitrile in coloured solutions	Dodecyl mercaptan	Conditions as in ref. 16	+ Acetic acid + isopropanol and titrated potentiometrically with $AgNO_3$ in ethanol–isopropanol,1 + 1	18
Acrylonitrile in air	Dodecyl mercaptan	40 l air passed through reagent in isopropanol at *ca.* − 70° taking *ca.* 20 min; KOH–alcohol then added; 4 min reaction	+ Acetic acid + I_2–KI equivalent to original mercaptan; unused iodine determined spectrophotometrically	19
Acrylonitrile	Mercapto-acetate (Na)	In methanol, + reagent; refluxed 30 sec–2 min	+ NH_4OH + NH_4Cl + Na_2SO_3 and titrated with Hg(II) acetate to thiofluorescein end-point (disappearance of blue)	20
Acrylonitrile		(Modification of method	of ref. 16)	21
Acrylonitrile in waste waters (> 1 g/l)	Thioglycol		Unreacted thioglycol determined iodometrically	22
Acrylonitrile	Mercapto-acetate	Sample + mercapto-acetic acid in 96% ethanol + Na_2CO_3 in ethanol–water; 2 min	+ HCl and back-titrated with iodine	23

butanol, saturated with water; visualisation then followed by spraying with ammoniacal silver nitrate solution which yields yellow spots, turning grey. Quantitative determination may be possible by comparing with the spots from known amounts of nitrile. Thiede and Franzen[26] also have used thiourea for detecting acrylonitrile in paper chromatography.

(*e*) *Addition of Alcohols*

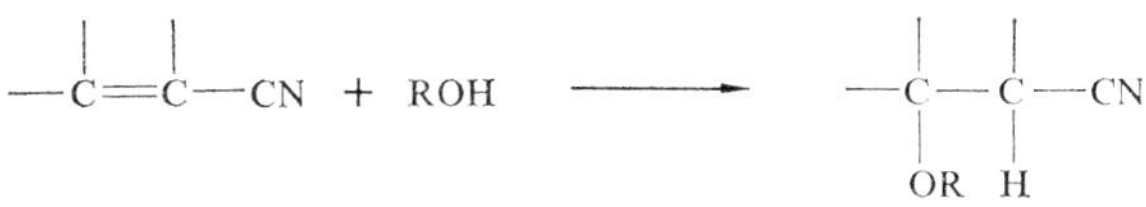

(3.8)

Two examples of the adaptation of this reaction to indirect determination may be quoted. Davis and Wiedeman[27] found that acrylonitrile was too volatile for convenient determination by alkaline hydrolysis to ammonia. They thus left the sample with sodium–ethanol for 1 hr, whereby cyanoethylation took place with formation of the involatile compound C_2H_5O—CH_2—CH_2—CN. Alkaline hydrolysis could then be carried out without losses.

Analysis of a mixture of acrylonitrile and 1-cyano-1,3-butadiene has been rendered possible by utilising reaction with an alcohol.[17] The sample was treated with potassium hydroxide–isopropanol for 45 min; under these conditions, acrylonitrile was cyanoalkylated. Unreacted 1-cyano-1,3-butadiene was then determined by the mercaptan method as was the sum of both unsaturated nitriles in a separate procedure (see p. 42). The amount of acrylonitrile was obtained by difference.

(*f*) *Addition of Bromine*

α,β-unsaturated carbonyl compounds, esters, acids, and nitriles generally add on halogens only slowly; satisfactory methods for their determination, based on this reaction, are few. Two examples are quoted here, both for determining a more reactive *cis*-isomer in the presence of the corresponding *trans*-isomer. Thus Buděšinský and Vaníčkova[28] determined *cis*-β-methoxy-α-ethoxymethylacrylonitrile in the presence of the *trans* compound by treating with a bromine reagent in acetic acid containing some pyridine and mercuric acetate as catalyst; reaction time was only 2 min and unused reagent was estimated by adding iodide and water and titrating with thiosulphate. Sterescu *et al.*(15) used the same method in analyses of nitrile mixtures in order to determine *cis*-α-(methoxymethylene)-β-methoxypropionitrile in the presence of the *trans* isomer and other nitriles.

(*g*) *Reaction with Ozone*

In their work on quantitative titration with an ozone–oxygen gaseous reagent, Boer and Kooyman(29) included the example of acrylonitrile. A constant current of oxygen containing a constant proportion of ozone is generated electrolytically from dilute sulphuric acid. The relation between duration of flow and amount of ozone is established by passing the gas mixture for measured times through potassium iodide solution and titrating the liberated iodine with thiosulphate. The standardised ozone–oxygen stream is then passed through a solution of the sample in chloroform; the time is measured to the end-point of decoloration of a dissolved indicator dye which is attacked after reaction with the sample is complete. The method is, of course, unselective since olefines of various types react to form ozonides.

(*h*) *Oxidation with Permanganate–Periodate*

Dal Nogare *et al.*(30) have determined acrylonitrile in distillates from polymers by adding sulphuric acid and periodic acid(3, 9) and titrating with permanganate at 0° to the first pink colour. Evidently the olefinic bond is converted to a 1,2-glycol which is then further oxidised by the periodic acid:

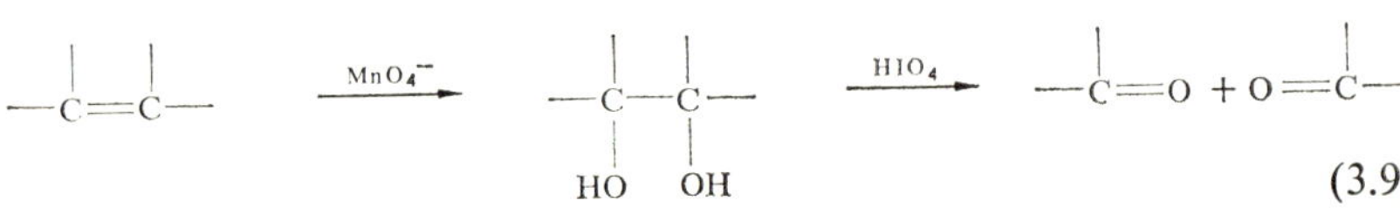

(3.9)

This simple method does not appear to have been tried out on other unsaturated nitriles.

(*i*) *Diels–Alder Reaction*

Tetracyanoethylene has been employed by Ozolins and Schenk(31) to determine many dienes (3.10).

Excess reagent was used and then back-titrated with standard cyclopentadiene in absolute ethanol. For this determination of the unused unsaturated nitrile, phenanthrene in benzene solution was used as a warning

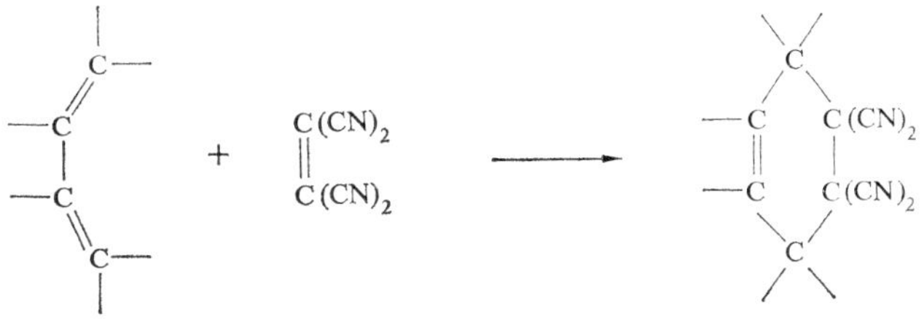

(3.10)

indicator; when the red-violet colour disappeared, the real indicator, a methylene dichloride solution of pentamethylbenzene, was added and titration was continued to the disappearance of the red colour. (Pentamethylbenzene cannot be added earlier during the titration because it forms so stable a complex with the tetracyanoethylene that it is decomposed only slowly by the cyclopentadiene.) The authors also carried out a photometric titration at 525 nm.

2. Compounds Containing the —CH_2CN or =CHCN Group

So-called "active" methylene and methine groups take part in a number of reactions, mostly in basic media, so that the first reaction stage is probably formation of a carbanion:

$$\begin{aligned} -CH_2X + OH^- &\rightleftharpoons -\bar{C}H-X + H_2O \\ =CHX + OH^- &\rightleftharpoons =\bar{C}-X + H_2O \end{aligned} \qquad (3.11)$$

Some of these reactions yield coloured products and are therefore adaptable to detection and eventually to quantitative colorimetric determination of compounds containing these groupings.

Some well-known colour reactions of this type are mentioned here. The cyano group is less activating than the carbonyl and nitro groups, for example. Consequently compounds containing only the —CH_2CN or =CHCN group may not always give a convincing response. Enhanced activation through a second cyano group or another group, such as the carbonyl or nitro group mentioned above or an aromatic nucleus, usually leads to a positive test.

(*a*) *Janovský Reaction with* m-*Dinitro Compounds and Alkali*

The first stage in this reaction is evidently attack of the carbanion of a free *p*-(or *o*-) position to one of the nitro groups (3.12).

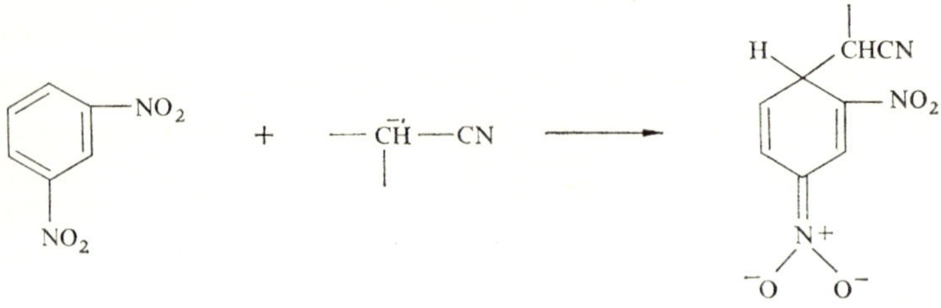

(3.12)

Janovský first described this reaction in 1886.[32] Ketones were used as the methylene component and it was not until the work of Reissert[33] that compounds containing activating groups other than the carbonyl group were found to participate. Canbäck[34] quotes, for example, benzyl cyanide, acetonitrile, and ethyl cyanoacetate, reacting with *m*-dinitrobenzene–alkali hydroxides to yield colours with absorption maxima in the 510–515 nm range and with molar absorption coefficients of *ca.* 15,000, 10,000 and 7000 respectively.

There are no firmly established conditions in use for carrying out this test. Alkali concentrations range from *ca.* 5 to 15% in water. *m*-Dinitrobenzene appears to give the most intense colours, and it is used in concentrations of a few percent in aqueous alcohol. Colour usually develops in the cold, but gentle warming may be necessary with less active methylene groups.

The colour reaction has been adapted to quantitative determination of phenylacetonitrile. Novotný[35] determined this compound in phenyl cyclohexylacetonitrile by dissolving the sample in 96% ethanol, adding saturated alcoholic picric acid solution, and then 20% alcoholic sodium hydroxide. The absorbance measurements were carried out at 530 nm. Ashworth and Schupp[36] used *m*-dinitrobenzene and potassium hydroxide, working in methanol–water (1 + 1) as solvent. With a reaction time of 22 min at 50°, Beer's law was found to hold for measurements at 425 nm on amounts up to 7 μg nitrile.

(*b*) *Reaction with Quinones*

Various initial reactions are possible between quinones and active methylene groups. The latter may attack the quinone at a —CH= group; they may attack at a carbon atom carrying a halogen or other group, ultimately with expulsion of this group; or they may add across the conjugated system (or across both ene–one systems of benzoquinone).

An early example of analytical application of reaction(s) with quinones is the test of Ehrlich and Herter[37] published in 1904. This depends on colour formation with 1,2-naphthoquinone-4-sulphonic acid in alkaline solution (sodium carbonate). Amongst their tabulated examples is cyanoacetic acid, stated to yield a red colour at first, turning red–purple after 2 min, red-violet on heating, and yellow on acidification with acetic acid. It is quoted by Feigl[38] as a test for active methylene and amino groups; he mentions that a violet colour is obtained with compounds containing the $—CH_2CN$ group, but gives no specific example nor information about sensitivity for cyano compounds. In the test, the sample is treated with a saturated solution of the reagent (sodium salt) and the solution is made faintly alkaline with alkali hydroxide. The first reaction is formulated with displacement of the $—SO_3^{(-)}$ group (3.13).

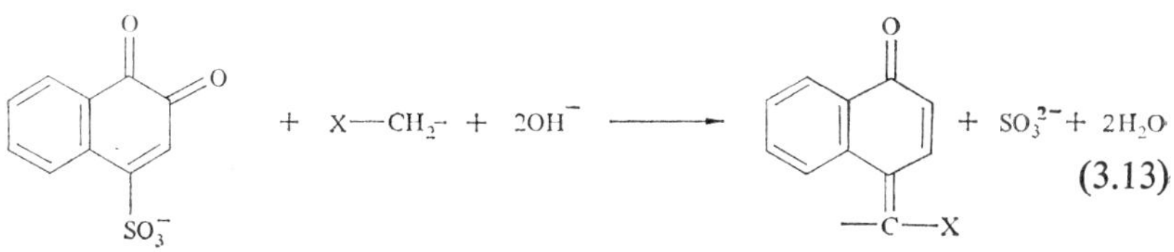

(3.13)

Saarivirta and Virtanen[39] have adapted the reaction to quantitative determination of phenylacetonitrile. An aqueous extract of the sample was allowed to react with the reagent for 4 min at 97–98°. Sodium hydroxide was then added, the mixture left for 20 min at room temperature, and the brown-red colour evaluated colorimetrically with a green filter.

Colour reactions with other quinones are mentioned in the literature. Thus Kesting[40] observed blue colours when malononitrile was treated with benzoquinone or 1,4-naphthoquinone in alcoholic solution and red with 1,2-naphthoquinone. He studied the influence of acid concentration and utilised differences in the rate of colour formation to detect small differences in the pH value of the solution. A few years later, in 1931, Craven[41] commented on the colour reaction between ethyl cyanoacetate and certain quinones, such as *p*-benzoquinone, *o*-toluquinone, 1,4-naphthoquinone, thymoquinone, and chloranil, in the presence of excess alcoholic ammonium hydroxide. The initial blue-violet colour changed rapidly through blue, green to reddish brown. Craven proposed this as a test for quinones which possess a labile hydrogen or halogen atom next to the —C=O group (thus 1,2-naphthoquinone, anthraquinone, and phenanthraquinone do not react). The test could clearly be applied in the reverse sense to detect ethyl cyanoacetate and other compounds, including nitriles having an active methylene group. Wood *et al.*[42] investigated the reaction further. They treated *p*-benzoquinone with cyanoacetic acid in alcohol–water–ammonium hydroxide, obtaining a purple-red precipitate after various colour changes in solution. Elemental analysis on this product indicated that two molecules of ester had evidently added on to the quinone, but without elimination of water or ethanol. Acid hydrolysis of the product, as well as of that obtained under similar conditions with malononitrile and with cyanoacetamide, yielded 2,5-dihydroxybenzenediacetic acid (3.14). Evidently two molecules of the active methylene component

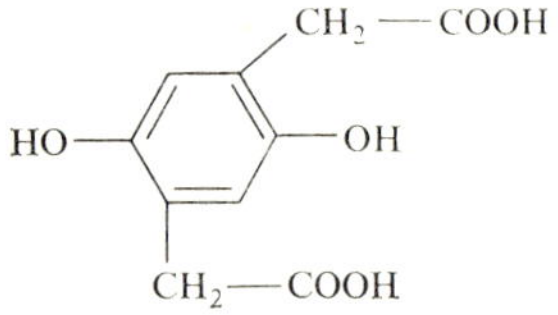

(3.14)

are added across each ene–one system but the exact nature of the coloured product(s) is unclear. Hess and Sullivan[43] noted that acetonitrile yields a red colour on shaking with benzoquinone–chloroform, and this could serve as a test. Considerable work has been done, especially by L. I. Smith and co-workers,[44] on the reaction between compounds containing an active methylene group and substituted benzoquinones; the comparative unavailability of these quinones renders small the potential value of the reactions, where they yield colours, as tests.

There appears to have been no attempt to adapt these colour reactions, in particular those with simpler quinones, to the quantitative colorimetric evaluation of compounds containing a —CH_2CN group. Gonter and Petty,[45] however, have been able to determine 1,4-naphthoquinone in phthalic anhydride through absorbance measurements at 583 nm after reaction with malononitrile in alkaline aqueous or alcoholic solution. They tried out other compounds in place of malononitrile, including other nitriles, and found that cyanoacetic acid yielded comparable absorbance values.

(c) *Reaction with Ketones*

Schenk and Finken[46] proposed a test for malononitrile, namely, the red colour obtained on shaking with fluorenone in alcoholic solution in the presence of a base such as ammonia or diethylamine (3.15).

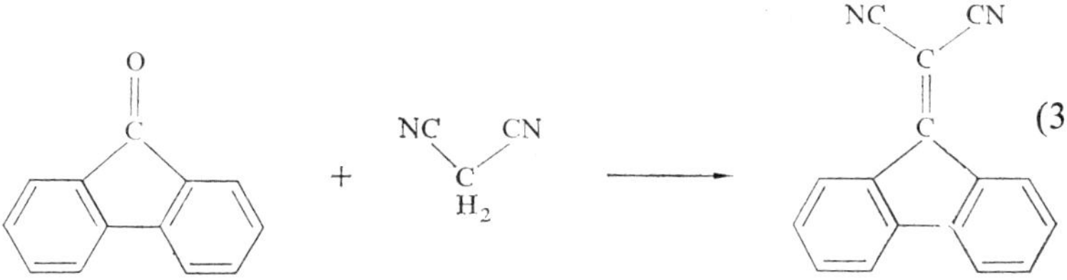

(3.15)

This appears neither to have been tested on other nitriles containing an active methylene group, nor worked out quantitatively.

(d) *Ehrlich–Sachs Reaction with* p-*Nitrosoalkylanilines*

This colour test is based on the preparative reactions of Ehrlich and co-workers, notably Sachs.[47] It is carried out by adding a concentrated solution of a base (sodium phosphate or potassium cyanide, for example, or pyridine) to the hot alcoholic solution of the sample and reagent. Colour develops on brief further heating.

Instead of the *p*-nitroso compound, the corresponding *p*-amino compound may be used in the presence of an oxidising agent. Thus Warfield[48] used ferricyanide. In his test, the sample is mixed with a solution of 1-amino-4-dimethylaminobenzene and sodium carbonate in water and a drop of 10% aqueous sodium ferricyanide is added. The only compound class containing a cyano group which Warfield cites is the $ArCOCH_2CN$ class; this yields a red–violet colour. Other oxidising agents may be used, e.g., persulphate, as suggested by Warfield.

Quantitative application of this reaction to compounds which possess a $—CH_2—CN$ group do not appear to be known.

(e) *Legal's Reaction with Nitroprusside–Alkali*

This test is known principally for methyl ketones but is given by other compound classes which contain an active methylene group. In Feigl's procedure[49] a drop of the sample solution is mixed with a drop of 5% sodium nitroprusside and a drop of 30% sodium hydroxide. After a short time, during which a slight colour usually develops, one or two drops of glacial acetic acid are added. A red or blue colour is yielded. Ethyl cyanoacetate is the only cyano compound quoted, without details of sensitivity.

It is believed that the nitroso group in the nitroprusside anion reacts with the active methylene group to yield an isonitroso compound (3.16).

$$—NO + —CH_2— \longrightarrow —\overset{|}{C}H—\overset{|}{N}—OH \qquad (3.16)$$

This then replaces the nitroso group in the complex. At the same time Fe(III) is reduced to Fe(II) so that the anion has 4- charge:

$$[Fe(CN)_5NO]^{2-} + —CH_2CN + 2OH^- \longrightarrow 2H_2O + [Fe(CN)_5ON{=}\underset{|}{C}—CN]^{4-} \qquad (3.17)$$

As with (*c*), there seems to have been no quantitative colorimetric application to the determination of cyano compounds.

(*f*) *Reaction with Diazonium Salts*

Compounds containing active methylene or methine groups have been detected and determined through coupling with diazonium salts. Some examples of the application of this to nitriles are given below (3.18).

$$R—\underset{CN}{\overset{|}{C}H} + [Ar—N{\equiv}N]^+ \longrightarrow R—\underset{CN}{\overset{|}{C}}—N{=}N—Ar— + H^+ \qquad (3.18)$$

Thus Lipton and co-workers[50, 51] identified cyanoacetic acid after paper chromatographic separation by spraying with diazotised sulphanilic acid and sodium carbonate, which gave orange-pink zones; or with diazotised *p*-nitroaniline, then yielding blue spots.

De Maldé[52] determined *cis*-1-cyano-1,3-butadiene by coupling with excess *p*-nitrobenzenediazonium salt in acetic acid–acetate buffer. After 15–30 hr reaction in the dark, unused diazonium salt was back-titrated with β-naphthol. Sievert *et al.*[53] developed a colorimetric method for determining cyanoacetic acid formed *in vitro* from β-aminopropionitrile in liver homogenates of various species; it was based on the orange colour yielded with diazotised sulphanilic acid in the presence of sodium carbonate, and enabled 1–7 μg amounts of the cyanoacetic acid to be determined. Lovelady[54] improved the method for determination of cyanoacetic acid in blood plasma. He replaced the sodium carbonate by sodium hydroxide, so that a stable colour was formed after 6 minutes and evaluated at 490 nm; amounts of 0·1–1 μg cyanoacetic acid could thus be estimated.

(*g*) *Reaction with Nitrosyl Chloride*

Perrot[55] has prepared derivatives from compounds having the $—CH_2—CN$ group by treatment with nitrosyl chloride. It was applied to aromatic examples where Ar = phenyl, substituted phenyl, or naphthyl (3.19).

$$\text{Ar—CH}_2\text{—CN} + \text{NOCl} \longrightarrow \text{Ar—}\underset{\substack{\| \\ \text{N—OH}}}{\text{C}}\text{—CN} + \text{HCl} \qquad (3.19)$$

These cyanooximes were also esterified, and melting-points were quoted for benzoates, *p*-nitrobenzoates, benzenesulphonates and *p*-toluenesulphonates as well.

(*h*) *Titration as Acids*

Compounds possessing active methylene groups may often be titrated as acids. Both Fritz and co-workers and Streuli have carried out such titrations in non-aqueous solution. Thus Fritz[56] titrated enols (including cyanoacetamide, ethyl cyanoacetate and malononitrile) in dimethylformamide with sodium ethoxide in benzene–methanol. Azo violet was a good indicator for the last-named and could be used also for the ester; cyanoacetamide was best titrated in ethylenediamine solution, using *o*-nitroaniline as indicator. Fritz and Yamamura[57] titrated enols in acetone with triethylbutylammonium hydroxide in benzene–methanol and potentiometric end-point indication; their examples included cyanoacetamide and malononitrile. Streuli,[58] in a comparison of relative acidities in pyridine and water, titrated many weak acids potentiometrically with tetrabutylammonium hydroxide. Cyanoacetamide, cyanamide and dicyanodiamide were titrated and it was possible to titrate each of the last two in the presence of the other; cyanamide is a much stronger acid (several powers of ten). (See also below.)

(*i*) *Reaction with Grignard Reagent* (*Methyl Magnesium Iodide*)

The determination of active hydrogen, based on measuring the methane evolved by reaction with methyl magnesium iodide, is a classical method of quantitative analysis and structure elucidation.

$$XH + CH_3MgI \longrightarrow XMgI + CH_4 \qquad (3.20)$$

Much work has been done on compounds which contain enolisable hydrogen in the structure $Y—\overset{|}{C}H—$, where Y is an activating group such as —CO—, —CN, $—NO_2$, etc. Activation by a single group of this type is evidently generally inadequate to lead to methane production. Two or more activating groups are necessary, but even then the equivalent of one active hydrogen may not be attained. There are few examples of the analysis of nitriles. Zaugg and Horrom(59) report 59% active hydrogen in diphenylacetonitrile in 5 min at 98°; and 12% active hydrogen with phenyl cyclohexylacetonitrile under the same conditions (in xylene solvent). McAlpine and Ongley(60) found almost one active hydrogen (97% in fact) in ethyl cyanoacetate in 5 min at 170°; phenylacetonitrile yielded only 59% under the same conditions.

(*j*) *Reaction with Lithium Aluminium Hydride*

This reaction was developed in the late forties as an alternative to methyl magnesium iodide for determining active hydrogen. Hydrogen is evolved according to:

$$4XH + LiAlH_4 \longrightarrow 4H_2 + LiX + AlX_3 \qquad (3.21)$$

The same considerations apply as under (*i*), hydrogen evolution taking place only when more than one activating group is present. Zaugg and Horrom(59) worked on the same examples as in (*i*). In di-n-butyl ether, diphenylacetonitrile yielded 47–48% active hydrogen under conditions ranging from 1 min at 98° or 20 min at 26° to 20 min at 98°. The phenyl cyclohexylacetonitrile showed only 6% active hydrogen under the same conditions.

3. Compounds Containing the —NH— or NH_2 Group Attached to —CN

Cyanamide and dicyanodiamide are important examples of compounds which contain this structural feature. Their simple formulae do not, in fact, always account for observed data. Thus the Raman spectrum of cyanamide indicates the existence of the tautomeric form NH=C=NH (3.22).

$$H_2N-C\equiv N \rightleftharpoons HN=C=NH \qquad (3.22)$$

Its formation of a dihydrochloride[61] can be explained better on the basis of the diimide structure (3.23).

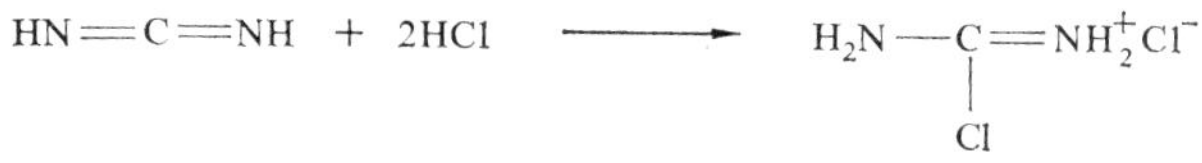

(3.23)

Hughes[62] has proposed a resonance hybrid of three structures (3.24) for dicyanodiamide, based on crystal structure data:

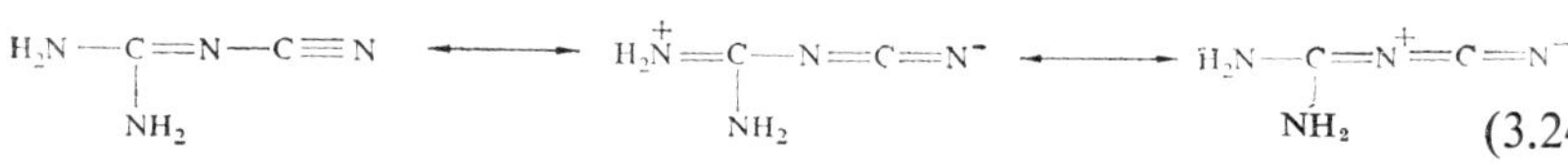

(3.24)

A discussion of this problem of tautomer and resonance structures lies outside the scope of this analytical monograph. Chemical analytical methods are most simply regarded from the point of view of the classically written structures. An approximate classification of chemical methods is given here.

(*a*) *Methods Based on the Acidic Nature of the H Atom*(*s*)

The strongly electron-withdrawing cyano group confers acidic properties on the —NH— or —NH_2 group linked to it. Although the values in the literature vary, it appears that the pK_A value for dissociation of the first hydrogen atom in cyanamide is about 1 (Soloway and Lipschitz[63] quote 1·1 and Grube and Motz[64] −0·36); that of the second is much higher, about 10 (Kameyama[65]). Salts in which both hydrogen atoms have been replaced, e.g. calcium cyanamide, are well known. Dicyanodiamide is an appreciably weaker acid, with a pK_A value in the region of 13–14 (Kameyama,[65] Grube and Krüger[66]).

The acidic properties of both compounds have been utilised in analysis. Thus Streuli[58] titrated each in the presence of the other, in pyridine solution, using tetrabutylammonium hydroxide and potentiometric end-point indication.

(b) Formation of Silver Salts

Better known are analytical methods based on formation of metal derivatives, chiefly with silver, but also with copper(II) and lead(II).

The reaction with silver ion

$$H_2N{-}CN + 2Ag^+ \longrightarrow Ag_2N{-}CN + 2H^+ \qquad (3.25)$$

yields a yellow product. This has been taken as a test for cyanamide, e.g by Korinfskii(67) and by Beeling and Laabs(68). Milks and Janes(69) and Knappe and Rohdewald(70) have used, amongst others, an ammoniacal spray reagent for detecting urea derivatives on paper chromatograms and thus visualised cyanamide through the yellow colour.

Quantitative argentometric determination of cyanamide dates back to 1905.(71) Most procedures have been concerned with analyses of calcium cyanamide manures and detailed conditions have been worked out for determining calcium cyanamide in the presence of commonly occurring impurities such as dicyanodiamide or urea. A selection of the fundamental procedures is quoted here. They are based on one of two principles:

(*i*) *Determination of the amount of Ag^+ used.* Shinozaki(72) titrated the sodium salt of cyanamide potentiometrically with silver nitrate; and Takei and Kato(73) titrated directly a solution of cyanamide in acetone containing ammonium hydroxide with silver nitrate reagent, using malachite green or methyl green as indicator. Apart from these examples, it appears that only indirect titration procedures have been used, precipitating from a weakly ammoniacal solution (the silver derivative of dicyanodiamide is much more soluble in this medium) with silver reagent in excess and back-titrating with thiocyanate after having filtered off the silver cyanamide. The original procedure of Perotti(71) was based on this principle, and some others who retained it with slight modifications of detail. In connection with the above-mentioned problem of calcium cyanamide analysis we include: Kappen,(74) Grube and Krüger,(75) Morrell and Burgen,(76) Yamazoe and Imai,(77) Capitani and Gambelli,(78) and Kramareva and Shul'man.(79)

(*ii*) *Separation and determination of the precipitate.* The determination of the precipitate has been accomplished in several ways:

1. It is dissolved in nitric acid and its silver content is determined by titration with thiocyanate; e.g. by Raida,(80) Pinck(81), and by Inaba

and Yangaisawa.[82] Yamada and Sakai[83] used this also for quantitative determination of spots of cyanamide on paper chromatograms which had been visualised with a silver reagent.

2. It is suspended in water and ammonium chloride, and a measured amount of standard sulphuric acid is added; after shaking, excess acid is back-titrated with alkali to methyl orange end-point (Nanussi).[84]

3. Through determination of nitrogen content with the Kjeldahl method. This is the classical method, used by many of the earlier workers in the 1907–20 period. Kühling,[85] Caro,[86] Stutzer and Söll,[87] and Hager and Kern[88] may be mentioned. Precipitation was often from an ammonium acetate-containing solution and supporters of this method claimed that it was independent of variations in the composition of the precipitate, such as those due to co-precipitated calcium carbide. In a study of the alkaline hydrolysis of cyanamide, Buchanan and Barsky[89] also determined the cyanamide by precipitation from ammoniacal solution, followed by Kjeldahl digestion. This is possibly the last reference to this somewhat laborious method (1930).

(*c*) *Formation of Other Metal Salts*

Beeling and Laabs[68] have detected small amounts of cyanamide through the formation of yellow lead cyanamide, PbN–CN. The solution to be tested was treated with ammonium hydroxide and a little lead hydroxide; the white suspension turned yellow slowly when cyanamide was present.

Nabiev *et al.*[90] gave two methods for the determination of cyanamide which depend on formation of the copper(II) derivative. In one, the volume of the CuN–CN precipitate from addition of cupric sulphate was measured after 2 hours; in the other, the sample + cupric sulphate was titrated with sulphuric acid to the disappearance of the black precipitate, or to the pink colour of added methyl orange indicator.

Methods depending on the formation of a silver derivative are also important for dicyanodiamide. Most methods have been concerned with the detection or determination in calcium cyanamide and the experimental conditions have been adjusted so as to permit either to be detected or determined in the presence of the other. The silver derivative of dicyanodiamide is more poorly soluble in nitric acid but more easily soluble in ammonium hydroxide than that of cyanamide. Thus Caro[86] precipitated first cyanamide in ammoniacal solution with silver acetate (see above), expelled ammonia from the filtrate by heating with alkali, and then precipitated the silver derivative of dicyanodiamide which was determined by conversion into ammonia through Kjeldahl digestion. Beeling and Laabs[68] recently mentioned the silver test by adding dilute nitric acid and then silver nitrate; formation of fine crystals and then a precipitate gives a positive test.

A more extensively used quantitative method for dicyanodiamide appears to involve precipitation with silver ions in the presence of picric acid, yielding a product formulated as $C_6H_2(NO_2)_3OAg{\cdot}C_2H_4N_4$. Harger[91] published the method in 1920 for determining dicyanodiamide in cyanamide and mixed fertilisers. An aliquot of the sample solution is treated with excess 5% aqueous silver nitrate and a large excess of saturated aqueous picric acid solution. After standing for 30 min in ice-water, the precipitate is filtered and determined gravimetrically, correcting for the solubility of the precipitate. Korinfskii[67] used a similar method, determining the precipitate gravimetrically and also dissolving in nitric acid and titrating the solution with thiocyanate. Inaba[92] has published work on a detailed study of Harger's procedure, suggesting also the use of excess silver ion and determination of the unused amount in the filtrate through titration with thiocyanate. Capitani and Gambelli[78] have worked on the argentometric determination of cyanamide and dicyanodiamide in mixtures of the two; they, too, employed the silver ion–picric acid method, with saturated picric acid solution. After leaving for 20 min at *ca.* 0° they filtered and also determined the excess silver ion in the filtrate by thiocyanate titration, potentiometrically or with ferric ion indicator. Johnson[93] modified Harger's method by treating an aliquot of the sample solution with nitric acid, sodium picrate, and excess standard silver nitrate at 5°. After 15 minutes at this temperature, the precipitate was filtered off and excess silver ion in the filtrate was titrated with thiocyanate. Johnson claimed that, under these conditions, a precipitate of composition $C_6H_2(NO_2)_3OAg{\cdot}C_2H_4N_4$ was formed which changes only slowly into the 1:1 compound at the low temperature used.

No work appears to have been done by analysts on the composition and structure of these picrates so that the classification of the reaction here is not justified with certainty. It is, however, a convenient place to mention it; moreover the 1:1 compound could equally well be formulated as a complex of picric acid and silver dicyanodiamide, $C_6H_2(NO_2)_3OH{\cdot}C_2H_3N_4Ag$.

(d) *Formation of the N—Cl Link*

Hofmann and Wünsch[94] have developed a number of colorimetric methods for cyanamide, dicyanodiamide, and related compounds; one of these depends on chlorination, evidently with formation of a —N—Cl link. The active halogen in this product may be detected in several ways. The authors proposed detection through the iodine yielded when iodide is added and also through the colour produced with benzidine; this latter test is based on the work of Reindel and Hoppe[95] who detected amines by chlorinating for 2 min and then treating with a 1 % solution of benzidine in 10 % acetic acid until maximum colour intensity was attained. Another method of detecting —N—Cl after chlorination is due to Ashworth and Bohnstedt[96] who used a cyanide/pyridine/1-phenyl-3-methyl-2-pyrazolinone-5 reagent. The active halogen yields chlorine cyanide which breaks the pyridine ring in alkaline solution, forming glutaconic dialdehyde monoenolate; this then gives an intensely coloured product with the pyrazolinone.

(e) *Miscellaneous Colour Reactions*

Both cyanamide and dicyanodiamide show numerous colour reactions, principally (but not exclusively) with cyanoferrate reagents such as nitroprusside and ferricyanide. The chemistry of these methods is often nuclear; it is, however, probably fair to say that a —NH_2 group participates, since many other compounds containing this group react similarly. Those reactions which have been adapted to both qualitative and quantitative analysis of cyanamide are tabulated here (Table 3.4). Analytically useful reactions of dicyanodiamide which probably involve an amino group, and also those in which the amidino group as a whole takes part are dealt with in Chapter 5, section 9; the present section is devoted only to reactions of the NH_2 or a —NH— group attached directly to the cyano group.

Some remarks may be appended here about the nature of these various colour reactions, although it is not intended to discuss this in detail.

The reactions with the various pentacyanoferrate complexes have been discussed in several of the publications cited in Table 3.4. It is significant that closely similar colours and spectra are obtained with all these reagents, suggesting a common end-product or at least closely related products. Buchanan and Barsky[107] found that cyanamide gave intense colours with ferrocyanide only after the latter had just been exposed to ultraviolet light but not if the exposed reagent had subsequently been left in the dark for an hour. Atmospheric oxygen evidently played no part in the changes since tests on aerated (with nitrogen) solutions yielded the same results. They postulated a photochemical equilibrium (3.26).

$$[Fe(CN)_6]^{4-} \xrightleftharpoons{h\nu} [Fe(CN)_5]^{3-} + CN^- \xrightleftharpoons{H_2N\cdot CN} [Fe(CN)_5\cdot H_2N\cdot CN]^{3-} \quad (3.26)$$

They observed colour directly with nitroprusside and noted that this colour formation was accelerated if the nitroprusside had likewise been exposed previously to ultraviolet radiation.

Baudisch[108] confirmed the phenomena with illuminated ferrocyanide but considered the changes to be as shown in formula (3.27). Baudisch

$$[Fe(CN)_6]^{4-} + H_2O \xrightleftharpoons{\text{Light}} [Fe(CN)_5OH]^{4-} + HCN$$

$$[Fe(CN)_5OH]^{4-} \xrightarrow{\text{air oxidation}} \text{intermediate} \xrightarrow{H_2N\cdot CN} \text{red complex} \quad (3.27)$$

found that cyanamide gave no colour with the pentacyanoaquoferrate (II) but also found that oxidation with air or hydrogen peroxide yielded a colour which was then removed by addition of the reducing agent cysteine. All these changes were reversible and Baudisch suggested (3.28)

$$[Fe(CN)_5H_2O]^{3-} + \text{oxidised nitrogen compounds} \longrightarrow [Fe(CN)_5X]^{3-} \quad (3.28)$$

where X = the organic component, probably containing a nitroso group.

Fearon[102] used (3.29) as a colour reagent for various nitrogen-contain-

$$[Fe(CN)_5NH_3]^{3-} \quad (3.29)$$

ing compounds, including cyanamide (in weakly alkaline solution at pH 8–9). This reagent was prepared from nitroprusside by treatment with conc. ammonium hydroxide and then oxidation in the air; this was found better than using an oxidising agent such as persulphate or iodine. Presumably the ammonia molecule is replaced in the colour-producing reaction by a nitrogen-containing molecule. Fearon suggested (3.30) where R= an alkyl group in amidines and =R—NH— in guanidines.

$$\left[Fe(CN)_5{\cdot}H_2N{-}\underset{\displaystyle R}{\underset{|}{C}}{=}NH\right]^{3-} \qquad (3.30)$$

Takimoto and Sawada[99] concluded that, in the nitroprusside–ferricyanide–base reaction with cyanamide, dicyanodiamide, etc., the anion yielded was (3.31) where X = an amidine.

$$[Fe(CN)_5X]^{3-} \qquad (3.31)$$

Buyske and Downing[104] also noted that cyanamide reacted with irradiated ferrocyanide but that long activation was necessary for a quantitative method to be possible. They therefore chose the ammine complex (3.29) for quantitative purposes. They observed that nitroprusside, too, yielded colour in alkaline solution (absorption maximum at 530 nm). They considered that nitroprusside might be partially hydrolysed in a photochemically catalysed reaction to yield (3.32) which in turn

$$[Fe(CN)_5H_2O]^{3-} \qquad (3.32)$$

reacts with the cyanamide. They found, however, that the absorbances produced with nitroprusside were only about one-quarter of those yielded with the ammine.

Summarising, it seems that the general opinion is that a coloured anion (3.31) is formed, where X is the compound under investigation or a derivative of it.

TABLE 3.4. COLOUR REACTIONS OF CYANAMIDE IN QUALITATIVE AND QUANTITATIVE ANALYSIS

Reagent	Purpose	Details	Reference
Nitroprusside–ferricyanide–alkali (a frequently used reagent is a 1:1:1 volume mixture of 10% aqueous solutions of Na salts and KOH)	Detection in PC*	Magenta colour	69
	Detection in PC	Red–violet	97
	Detection in PC		98
	Quantitative determination		99
	Detection in PC		100
	Detection in TLC	Purple	70
	Quantitative determination	NH_4OH as alkali; 5 min at 50°; 525 nm	101
Nitroprusside–hydrogen peroxide	Detection in PC	Violet	94
Pentacyanoammino-ferrates (3.29)	Test	Orange-red at pH 8–9	102
	Detection in PC		103
	Quantitative determination in urine	Absorbance at 530 nm	104
	Quantitative determination in soil and plants	Absorbance at 530 nm in Na_2CO_3–HCl, pH 10·5	105
	Quantitative determination in ginned cotton seed	Absorbance at 530 nm in carbonate buffer of pH 10·4	106
1,2-Naphthoquinone-4-sulphonate–alkali	Detection in PC	Orange–red after heating	69
N,N-Dimethylaminobenzaldehyde–HCl	Detection in PC	Yellow	69
	Detection in TLC	Inspected in light of 254 or 366 nm	70
α-Naphthol–hypohalite–alkali ("Sakaguchi" reagent)	Detection in TLC	Violet	70

* PC = paper chromatography.
TLC = thin layer chromatography.

1,2-Naphthoquinone-4-sulphonate has been mentioned already (p. 47) as a reagent for active methylene and for amino groups. The probable reaction (3.33) is replacement of the sulphonate group by =N—CN.

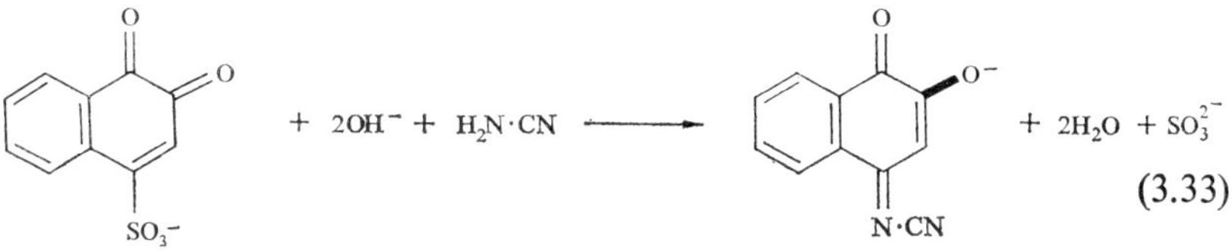

(3.33)

Dimethylaminobenzaldehyde evidently reacts with formation of an azomethine (3.34).

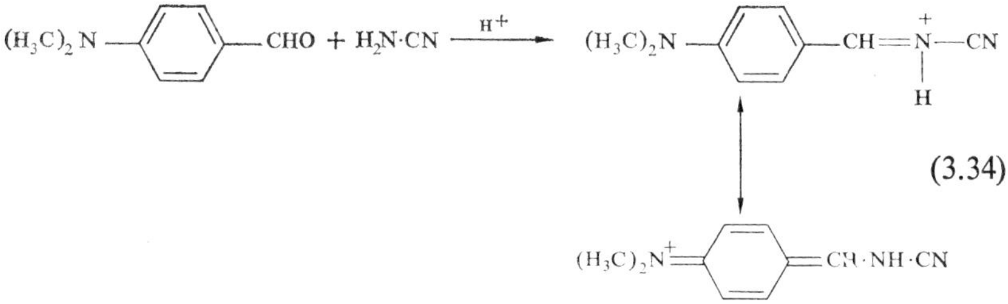

(3.34)

The "Sakaguchi" test[109] is for arginine in proteins and eqn. (3.34) probably involves reaction with the group shown in (3.35) since other

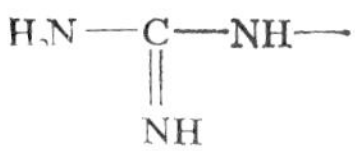

(3.35)

compounds containing this guanidyl group react also, e.g. dicyanodiamide (see below, p. 73). Cyanamide may react through initial dimerisation to dicyanodiamide or directly through the —NH_2 group. This does not appear to have been studied analytically.

(*f*) *Reactions as Bases*

The fact that cyanamide and dicyanodiamide form dihydrochlorides[61] raises the hope of determining them as bases. Cyanamide is evidently an extremely feeble base; Grube and Motz[64] found a pK_B value in water of about 15. It is thus probably too weak even to be titrated in acidic solvents such as glacial acetic acid. The author has found no reference to a titration of this sort. Dicyanodiamide is rather less weak—it contains the guanidino group (3.35) derived from the strong organic base guanidine.

Polaczek and Grzeszkiewicz[110] have been able to titrate it and also *p*-chlorophenyldicyanodiamide in acetic acid containing mercuric acetate, using perchloric acid in acetic acid as titrant. They determined the end-point potentiometrically or with crystal violet. They attributed the basic properties of these compounds to the diimide tautomeric form (3.36)

$$-NH-C\equiv N \rightleftharpoons -N=C=NH \qquad (3.36)$$

which then forms a mercuric acetate derivative—N=C=N—$HgOOCCH_3$. They claimed that the method should be applicable to any cyano compound which can yield the carbodiimide tautomer.

References

1. Brockway, C. E., *Anal. Chem.* **21**, 1207 (1949).
2. Terent'ev, A. P., Butskus, P. F., and Yashinskii, V. G., *Zh. Anal. Khim.* **9**, 162 (1954).
3. Critchfield, F. E., Funk, G. L., and Johnson, J. B., *Anal. Chem.* **28**, 76 (1956).
4. Terent'ev, A. P., Buzlanova, M. M., and Obtemperanskaya, S. I., *Zh. Anal. Khim.* **14**, 506 (1959).
5. Terent'ev, A. P., Buzlanova, M. M., Obtemperanskaya, S. I., and Volod'zko, V. E., *Vestn. Mosk. Univ., Ser. Khim.* 83 (1962); *Chem. Abs.* **56**, 2850 (1962); *Chem. Zbl.* **13**, 1698 (1964).
6. Belcher, R. and Fleet, B., *Talanta* **12**, 677 (1965).
7. Terent'ev, A. P., Obtemperanskaya, S. I., and Buzlanova, M. M., *Zavod. Lab.* **24**, 814 (1958).
8. Critchfield, F. E. and Johnson, J. B., *Anal. Chem.* **28**, 73 (1956).
9. Terent'ev, A. P. and Obtemperanskaya, S. I., *Zh. Anal. Khim.* **11**, 638 (1956).
10. Terent'ev, A. P., Obtemperanskaya, S. I., and Buzlanova, M. M., *Vestn. Mosk. Univ.*, 11 *Ser. Mat. Mekh., Astron., Fiz., Khim.* No. 1, 187 (1956); *Chem. Abs.* **51**, 11935 (1957).
11. Kostin, L. D. and Vidanova, V. A., *USSR Patent* 104,643, 25/1/57; *Chem. Abs.* **51**, 7246 (1957).
12. Terent'ev, A. P., Obtemperanskaya, S. I., and Buzlanova, M. M., *Zavod. Lab.* **24**, 157 (1958).
13. Obtemperanskaya, S. I., Terent'ev, A. P., and Buzlanova, M. M., *Zh. Anal. Khim.* **16**, 372 (1961).
14. Philipp, B., Bartels, U., and Hayme, H., *Faserforsch. Textiltech.* **12**, 581 (1961).
15. Sterescu, M., Aftalion, H., Ionescu, M., Cilianu, S., Rogozea, I., and Ioan, C., *Arch. Pharm.* **298**, 820 (1965).
16. Beesing, D. W., Tyler, W. P., Kurtz, D. M., and Harrison, S. A., *Anal. Chem.* **21**, 1073 (1949).
17. De Maldé, M., *Ann. Chim.* (*Rome*) **42**, 437 (1952).
18. Janz, G. J. and Duncan, N. E., *Anal. Chem.* **25**, 1410 (1953).

19. HASLAM, J. and NEWLANDS, G., *Analyst (London)* **80**, 50 (1955).
20. WROŃSKI, M., *Chem. Anal. (Warsaw)* **5**, 823 (1960).
21. MAJEWSKA, J., and URBANOWICZ, S., *Chem. Anal. (Warsaw)* **6**, 841 (1961).
22. KRAITSMAN, P. S. and CHEKHOVSKAYA, F. V., *Gig. i Sanit.* **30**, No. 6 57 (1965); *Z. anal. Chem.* **230**, 65 (1967).
23. KOVACS, I., *Munkavedelem* **12**, 23 (1966); *Chem. Abs.* **66**, 4904 (1967); also in *Magy. Kem. Folyoirat* **73**, 189 (1967); *Chem. Abs.* **67**, 723 (1967).
24. STĚPÁNEK, J. M. and ČERNÁ, V. M., *Analyst (London)* **83**, 345 (1958).
25. STĚPÁNEK, J. M., ČERNÁ, V. M., and PATKOVÁ, V. J., *Analyst (London)* **84**, 65 (1959).
26. THIEDE, H. and FRANZEN, E., *Wiss. Z. Martin Luther Univ., Halle-Wittenberg, Math.-Nat. Reihe* **14**, 177 (1965).
27. DAVIS, H. S. and WIEDEMAN, O. F., *Ind. Eng. Chem.* **37**, 482 (1945).
28. BUDĚŠINSKÝ, B. and VANÍČKOVA, E., *Česk. Farm.* **6**, 305 (1957).
29. BOER, H. and KOOYMAN, E. C., *Anal. Chim. Acta* **5**, 550 (1951).
30. DAL NOGARE, S., PERKINS, L. R., and HALE, A. H., *Anal. Chem.* **24**, 512 (1952).
31. OZOLINS, M. and SCHENK, G. H., *Anal. Chem.* **33**, 1035 (1961).
32. JANOVSKÝ, J. V., *Chem. Ber.* **19**, 2158 (1886).
33. REISSERT, A., *Chem. Ber.* **37**, 831 (1904).
34. CANBÄCK, T., *Svensk Farm. Tids.* **54**, 1201 (1950).
35. NOVOTNÝ, B., *Czechoslovak Patent* 101,926 (15/12/61); *Chem. Abs.* **58**, 10737 (1963).
36. ASHWORTH, M. R. F. and SCHUPP, R., *Mikrochim. Acta* 366 (1967).
37. EHRLICH, P. and HERTER, C. A., *Z. Physiol. Chem.* **41**, 37 (1904).
38. FEIGL, F., "*Spot Tests in Organic Analysis*", 7th English Edn., Elsevier Pub. Co. 1966, p. 153.
39. SAARIVIRTA, M. and VIRTANEN, A. I., *Acta Chem. Scand.* **17**, suppl. 1, 74 (1963).
40. KESTING, W., *Z. Angew. Chem.* **41**, 358, 745 (1938).
41. CRAVEN, R., *J. Chem. Soc.* 1605 (1931).
42. WOOD, J. H., COLBURN, C. S., COX, L., and GARLAND, H. C., *J. Am. Chem. Soc.* **66**, 1540 (1944).
43. HESS, W. C. and SULLIVAN, M. X., *J. Biol. Chem.* **99**, 96 (1933).
44. SMITH, L. I. *et al.*, for example: *J. Am. Chem. Soc.* **76**, 3651 (1950); *J. Org. Chem.* **25**, 832 (1950).
45. GONTER, C. E. and PETTY, J. J., *Anal. Chem.* **35**, 663 (1963).
46. SCHENK, R. and FINKEN, H., *Ann.* **462**, 269 (1928).
47. EHRLICH, P. and SACHS, F., *Chem. Ber.* **32**, 2341 (1899); see also *Chem. Ber.* **33**, 959 (1900) and **34**, 118,494 (1901).
48. WARFIELD, P. F., *Anal. Chem.* **24**, 890 (1952).
49. FEIGL, F., "*Spot Tests in Organic Analysis*", 7th English edn., Elsevier Pub. Co. p. 208 (1966).
50. LIPTON, S. H., LALICH, J. J., and STRONG, F. M., *J. Am. Chem. Soc.* **80**, 2022 (1958).
51. LIPTON, S. H., LALICH, J. J., GARBUTT, J. T., and STRONG, F. M., *J. Am. Chem. Soc.* **80**, 6594 (1958).
52. DE MALDÉ, M., *Ann. Chim. (Rome)* **42**, 431 (1952).
53. SIEVERT, H. W., LIPTON, S. H., and STRONG, F. M., *Arch. Biochem. Biophys.* **86**, 311 (1960).
54. LOVELADY, H. G., *Anal. Chem.* **34**, 1344 (1962).
55. PERROT, R., *Comptes Rendus*, **199**, 585 (1934).
56. FRITZ, J. S., *Anal. Chem.* **24**, 674 (1952).
57. FRITZ, J. S. and YAMAMURA, S. S., *Anal. Chem.* **29**, 1079 (1957).

58. Streuli, C. A., *Anal. Chem.* **32**, 407 (1960).
59. Zaugg, H. E. and Horrom, B. W., *Anal. Chem.* **20**, 1026 (1948).
60. McAlpine, I. M. and Ongley, P. U., *Anal. Chem.* **27**, 55 (1955).
61. Johnson, T. B. and Sprague, J. M., *J. Am. Chem. Soc.* **61**, 176 (1939).
62. Hughes, E. W., *J. Am. Chem. Soc.* **62**, 1258 (1940).
63. Soloway, S. and Lipschitz, A., *J. Org. Chem.* **23**, 613 (1958).
64. Grube, G. and Motz, G., *Z. Physik. Chem.* **118**, 145 (1925).
65. Kameyama, N., *Trans. Am. Electrochem. Soc.* **40**, 131 (1921); *J. Chem. Ind. (Japan)* **24**, 1263 (1921).
66. Grube, G. and Krüger, J., *Z. Physik. Chem.* **86**, 85 (1914).
67. Korinfskii, A. A., *Zavod. Lab.* **11**, 816 (1945).
68. Beeling, H. and Laabs, W., *Z. anal. Chem.* **215**, 35 (1966).
69. Milks, J. E. and Janes, R. H., *Anal. Chem.* **28**, 846 (1956).
70. Knappe, E. and Rohdewald, I., *Z. anal. Chem.* **223**, 174 (1966).
71. Perotti, R., *Gazz. Chim. Ital.* **35** (II), 228 (1905).
72. Shinozaki, H., *J. Soc. Chem. Ind. (Japan)* **36** (Suppl. Binding) 145 (1933).
73. Takei, S. and Kato, T., *Technol. Repts. Tôhoku Univ.* **18**, 159 (1954).
74. Kappen, H., *Landwirtschaftliche Versuchsstationen* **70**, 454 (1909); Beilstein, I. Ergänzungswerk I p. 78; *Z. anal. Chem.* **50**, 125 (1911).
75. Grube, G. and Krüger, J., *Z. Angew Chem.* **27**, 326 (1914).
76. Morrell, G. F. and Burgen, P., *J. Chem. Soc.* **105**, 576 (1914).
77. Yamazoe, F. and Imai, J., *Nippon Dojo-Hiryogaku Zasshi* **31**, 245 (1960).
78. Capitani, C. and Gambelli, G., *Chim. Ind. (Milan)* **35**, 890 (1960).
79. Kramareva, T. V. and Shul'man, V. M., *Zh. Anal. Khim.* **23**, 750 (1968).
80. Raida, H., *Z. Ges. Exptl. Med.* **31**, 215 (1923).
81. Pinck, L. A., *Ind. Eng. Chem.* **17**, 459 (1925).
82. Inaba, H. and Yanigasawa, D., *Japan Analyst* **3**, 196 (1954).
83. Yamada, T. and Sakai, Y., *Denki Kagaku (J. Electrochem. Soc. Japan)* **29**, 852 (1961).
84. Nanussi, A., *Giorn. Chim. Ind. Applicata* **5**, 168 (1923).
85. Kühling, O., *Chem. Ber.* **40**, 313 (1907).
86. Caro, N., *Z. Angew. Chem.* **23**, 2408 (1910).
87. Stutzer, A. and Söll, J., *Z. Angew. Chem.* **23**, 1874 (1910).
88. Hager, G. and Kern, J., *Z. Angew. Chem.* **29**, 309 (1916); **30**, 53 (1917).
89. Buchanan, G. H. and Barsky, G., *J. Am. Chem. Soc.* **52**, 198 (1930).
90. Nabiev, M. N., Matveev, M. A., and Shakirov, Yu. I., *Sotsiol. Sel'sk. Khoz. Uzbekistana* No. 8, 54 (1956); *Chem. Abs.* **53**, 12933 (1959).
91. Harger, R. N., *Ind. Eng. Chem.* **12**, 1107 (1920).
92. Inaba, H., *Japan Analyst* **3**, 107 (1954).
93. Johnson, E. B., *Ind. Eng. Chem.* **13**, 533 (1921).
94. Hofmann, E. and Wünsch, A., *Naturwissenschaften* **45**, 338 (1958).
95. Reindel, F. and Hoppe, W., *Naturwissenschaften* **40**, 221 (1953).
96. Ashworth, M. R. F. and Bohnstedt, G., *Talanta* **13**, 1631 (1966).
97. May, K., Rothe, O., and May, L., *Melliand. Textilber.* **40**, 899 (1959).
98. Takimoto, M., and Koeda, K., *Kogyo Kagaku Zasshi* **63**, 797 (1960); *Chem. Abs.* **56**, 6639 (1962); *Chem. Zbl.* 3925 (1962).
99. Takimoto, M. and Sawada, M., *J. Chem. Soc. Japan, Ind. Chem. Sect.* **63**, 967 (1960); *Chem. Zbl.* 3722 (1963).
100. Meckel, L. and Milster, H., *Textil-Rundschau* **16**, 593 (1961); **17**, 485 (1962).
101. Mushkin, Yu. I., *Zavod. Lab.* **33**, 296 (1967).
102. Fearon, W. R., *Analyst (London)* **71**, 562 (1946).

103. LIST, P. H., *Z. Physiol. Chem.* **303**, 27 (1956).
104. BUYSKE, D. A. and DOWNING, V., *Anal. Chem.* **32**, 1798 (1960).
105. ROTINI, O. T. and GALOPPINI, C., *Agrochimica (Pisa)* **10**, 9 (1965).
106. STELLER, W. A., FREDERICK, I. B., and MORGAN, P. W., *J. Agr. Food Chem.* **13**, 329 (1965).
107. BUCHANAN, G. H. and BARSKY, G., *Angew. Chem.* **44**, 383 (1931).
108. BAUDISCH, O., *Chem. Ber.* **68**, 773 (1935).
109. SAKAGUCHI, S., *J. Biochem. (Japan)* **5**, 25, 134, 140 (1925).
110. POLACZEK, L. and GRZESZKIEWICZ, A., *Chem. Anal. (Warsaw)* **9**, 1045 (1964).

CHAPTER 4

REACTIONS OF GROUPS SENSIBLY UNAFFECTED BY THE CYANO GROUP

1. Higher Aliphatic Nitriles

Tang and Kuo[1] demonstrated the presence in shale oil of nitriles with long straight chains; urea clathrate formation (and also chromatography) were the techniques used.

Iida *et al.*[2] also used urea adduct formation to separate straight chain nitriles (C_{12}–C_{15}) from a neutral Colorado shale oil distillate of b.p. 280–305°; hydrocarbons and ketones likewise formed adducts but were subsequently separated by column chromatography.

2. β, γ-Unsaturated Nitriles

A problem of long standing is quantitative determination of mixtures of isomeric unsaturated compounds containing an activating group such as =CO, —CN, —NO_2, or —Ar. It is known that so-called α,β-unsaturated carbonyl compounds, esters, nitriles, nitro compounds, etc., add on electrophilic reagents, such as bromine, only slowly; where the activating and the olefinic group are more separated, such as in the β,γ-isomers, this reactivity is less impaired and resembles that of an isolated olefine group. This difference in reactivity between α,β- and β,γ-isomers is, however, usually insufficiently large for the latter to react sensibly completely without the former having entered into reaction. Attempts have been made to develop kinetic methods for binary mixtures, using suitable reagents under appropriate conditions. Prominent among these reagents are bromine and iodine; excess was used and the unreacted amount was determined by back-titration with thiosulphate (after having added iodide in the case of bromine addition).

Sudborough and Thomas[3] appear to have been the first to refer to this difference in reactivity (of unsaturated carboxylic acids and esters) with halogens as a means of distinguishing α,β- from β,γ- or γ,δ-forms. In the 1920–40 period, several teams working on preparation of unsaturated nitriles and other compounds devised halogen reagents for this purpose, choosing conditions so as to yield as large a contrast as possible between the extent of reaction of the α,β- and the β,γ-isomers. Interpolation then gave an approximate value of the composition of a α,β–β,γ-mixture. Those principally active were Linstead and his co-workers in Britain, the Belgian school of Bruylants, Heim and others, and Delaby and co-workers in France. Linstead[(4)] first suggested dissolving both sample and bromine in carbon tetrachloride or chloroform; Linstead and May[(5)] then extended this to an iodine–potassium iodide aqueous reagent with the sample (in this case unsaturated acids) in saturated sodium bicarbonate solution; and an iodine–mercuric chloride–ethanol (iodine monochloride) reagent, using the sample in ethanol. Heim,[(6)] for example, dissolved the sample in chloroform and employed aqueous bromine–bromide in two-fold excess. All these methods are special analyses of particular binary mixtures and have no general application.

3. Aromatic Groups in Nitriles

Okhuma[(7)] quotes a test for phenylacetonitrile which depends on nitration with potassium nitrate–conc. sulphuric acid to form the 2,4-dinitro compound; after rendering the solution basic with ammonium hydroxide, the *m*-dinitro compound is extracted with chloroform, the solvent evaporated, and the residue treated with acetone and a few drops of sodium hydroxide solution. A red-violet colour (Janovský reaction) is given. The test is not specific, since it may be applied to any aromatic compounds which yield *m*-dinitro derivatives.

A quantitative example of the utilisation of a typical electrophilic substitution reaction is given by Fleszar[(8)] for the determination of *p*-aminobenzoylacetonitrile (4.1). Amongst other methods, such as

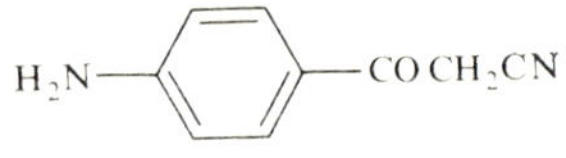

(4.1)

diazotisation of the amino group (see below under 8) and photometry at

328 nm, he used titration with bromate. Ethanol, potassium bromide, and 50% hydrochloric acid were added to an aliquot of a stock solution of the nitrile in *ca.* 1 N hydrochloric acid, and the solution was titrated with standard bromate to the permanent deflection (5 min) of the galvanometer in a potentiometric system consisting of a platinum and a calomel electrode. The method is, of course, available in principle for any sufficiently reactive aromatic nucleus.

4. Halogen Atoms in Trichloroacetonitrile

Lubatti and Harrison[9] determined this insecticide by passing it in a mixture with air and hydrogen peroxide through silica tubes containing platinum filaments at dull redness. The exit gases were absorbed in alkali, acetic acid was added, and the chloride ion was determined by titration with silver nitrate to chromate indicator.

5. Azo Group in Azobisisobutyronitrile

This compound and some of similar structure have been proposed as initiators in the polymerisation of methyl methacrylate and styrene.[10] Lada[11] determined it by heating at 98° and measuring the nitrogen evolved according to eqn. (4.2)

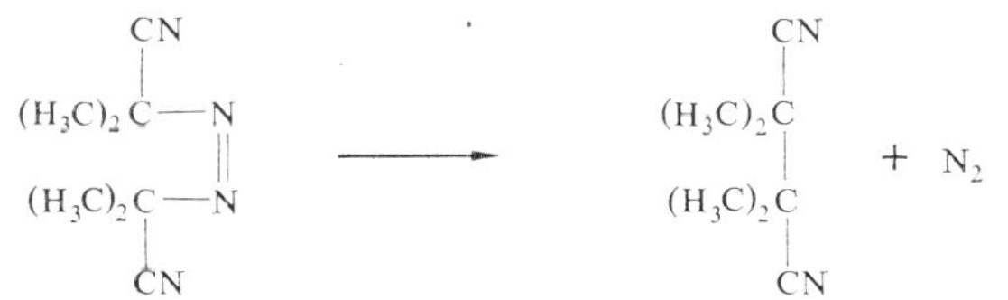

(4.2)

Polarographic methods have been used for quantitative determination. These are classified in a separate section (p. 125) but two examples may be given here also. Bobrova and Matveeva determined the 2,2′-azobisisobutyronitrile in 50% aqueous ethanol with tetra-n-butylammonium iodide as supporting electrolyte[12] or in 50–75% ethanol using lithium chloride.[13] A linear relation between concentration and diffusion current was found in the concentration range studied (1–10 μmole/l). Dmitrieva and Bezuglyi[14] determined it in polymers, using 92% methanol with tetraethylammonium iodide as supporting electrolyte or in benzene–methanol (1 + 4) plus lithium chloride or buffer mixtures. Again a linear relation was established between current and concentration. The two-electron change found evidently corresponds to reduction of the azo group as shown in eqn. (4.3, left to right).

$$-N{=}N- \quad + \; 2H^{+} \; + \; 2\varepsilon \quad \longleftrightarrow \quad -NH-NH- \qquad (4.3)$$

6. Hydrazo Group in 2,2′-Hydrazobisisobutyronitrile

This is the reaction product from (polarographic) reduction of the azo compound in the previous paragraph. McBride *et al.*[15] studied the oxidation with iodate of many hydrazine derivatives, including this hydrazo compound. They found a two-electron quantitative oxidation in 9 N hydrochloric or sulphuric acid in direct potentiometric titration with potassium iodate. Clearly, oxidation to the azo compound takes place (4.3, right to left).

7. Ester Group in Nitriles

Ester groups are in general much more easily hydrolysed than cyano groups. The usual saponification procedures may thus be applicable to the quantitative determination of esters which contain such a group. There appears to be no publication specially referring to an example of this sort in which the consumption of alkali reagent was measured, or in which the carboxylic acid reaction product was isolated and determined by a classical method, such as titration with alkali. Maros *et al.*,[16] however, quote ethyl phenylethylcyanoacetate among some examples of compounds which they determined by hydrolysis with $Ba(OH)_2$ to a product which is easily decarboxylated; this was followed by determination[17] of the carbon dioxide using a previously developed method (distillation into excess $Ba(OH)_2$ and back-titration with HCl to thymol blue):

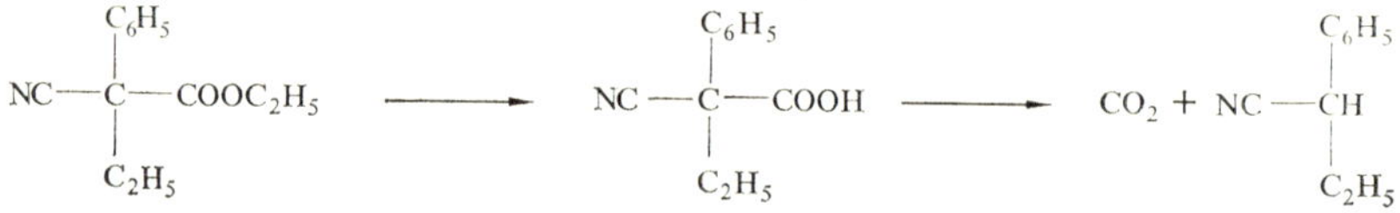

(4.4)

Presumably either hydrolysis of the cyano group is negligible or the acid formed through its hydrolysis does not decarboxylate so readily.

8. Amino Groups (not Directly Linked to a Cyano Group)

Cyano compounds containing an amino group possess basic properties which can be utilised for their determination. Thus Wagner and Kauffman[18] mention *N,N'*-bis(2-cyanoethyl)-2,5-dimethylpiperazine among some aromatic amines which they titrated in acetic acid, using perchloric acid–acetic acid and the so-called "high frequency" end-point indication. Streuli[19] has titrated some copolymers of acrylonitrile with bases such as unsaturated amines or unsaturated quaternary ammonium compounds; these were dissolved in nitromethane and formic acid added if necessary to achieve a clear solution; titrant was perchloric acid in dioxan and end-point indication was potentiometric. In an attempt to correlate structure with titration behaviour, Streuli[20] determined some pK_A values in nitromethane by potentiometric titration with perchloric acid. His examples included cyanoethyl compounds, e.g. 2-cyanoethylamine, bis-2-cyanoethylamine and tris-2-cyanoethylamine.

An example of a different sort is the determination of β-aminopropionitrile (2-cyanoethylamine) in mature legume seeds by Garbutt and Strong.[21] This is based on spectrophotometry of the reaction product at 640 nm with ninhydrin in n-butanol (20 min at *ca.* 100°, then cooled and NaOH added). Down to 50 ppm could be determined.

Fleszar[8] titrated *p*-aminobenzoylacetonitrile potentiometrically in dilute hydrochloric acid solution containing bromide; the titrant was sodium nitrite.

9. Amidino or Guanidino Group in Dicyanodiamide

Some chemical methods for detection or determination of dicyanodiamide have been mentioned already in Chapter 2 (addition to the cyano group) and Chapter 3 (probably reactions of the —NH-group linked to the cyano group). In Chapter 5 are discussed methods which depend on degradation of the molecule, whereby the cyano group remains intact. In the present section, chemical methods (mostly colorimetric) based on reactions of the amidino (4.5) or guanidino moieties (4.6) are given. The

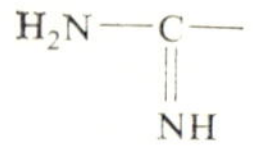

(4.5)

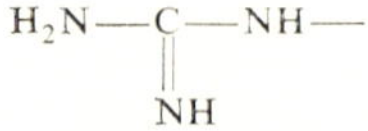

(4.6)

chemistry of the following reactions is not always clear but the following rough classification may be attempted into methods depending on:

(a) Reactions of an amino group, similar to those shown by this group in other compounds such as cyanamide (or even primary amines) and which are not necessarily amidino or guanidino compounds.

(b) Reactions probably of an amino group as part of the amidino or guanidino group and which evidently do not occur with other amino groups.

(c) Reactions in which two centres of the amidino or guanidino group participate.

(*a*) *Reactions of an Amino Group, not necessarily part of the Amidino or Guanidino Group*

Various alkaline nitroprusside reagents containing oxidising agents such as hydrogen peroxide or ferricyanide, yield colours with dicyanodiamide as with cyanamide (see Table 3.4) and have been utilised, especially for detection. Thus Hofmann and Wünsch[22] proposed a nitroprusside–hydrogen peroxide–alkali reagent for detection in paper chromatography (PC); it yields carmine red with dicyanodiamide, and violet with cyanamide. The nitroprusside–ferricyanide–alkali reagent has found extensive application: Milks and Janes[23] quote it for detection of dicyanodiamide in PC; the colour yielded (magenta) is the same as that from cyanamide. May *et al.*[24] mention red–violet as the colour from dicyanodiamide in PC-visualisation (red from cyanamide). Others who have made use of this colour reagent for detection in PC and TLC are: Takimoto and Koeda;[25] Milster and Meckel;[26] Woggon *et al.*;[27] Ardelt and Lange;[28] and Knappe and Rohdewald.[29] Takimoto and Sawada[30] developed a quantitative colorimetric method for determining amounts of dicyanodiamide of 5–50 μg/l with 1–2% error; the absorbance at 515 nm was measured.

The pentacyanoamminoferrate reagent (3.29) has been used by List[31] as a spray reagent for detecting dicyanodiamide (and cyanamide) in PC.

In the method for detection of cyanamide and dicyanodiamide by chlorination and subsequent treatment with iodide or with benzidine (p. 57),[22] it is, of course, possible that —NH—groups in dicyanodiamide other than that linked to the cyano group also react to yield —NCl—. This does not affect the issue.

There is conflicting information about two other colour reagents given in Table 3.4 when applied to dicyanodiamide. Thus Milks and Janes[23] state that it yields no colour with their reagent (dimethylaminobenzaldehyde in 1·2 N hydrochloric acid); but Korn and Woggon[32, 33] quote a spray reagent of dimethylaminobenzaldehyde–phosphoric acid–acetic acid–butanol for TLC of PVC stabilisers, including dicyanodiamide; further, Knappe and Rohdewald[29] used a reagent made up of the aldehyde in hydrochloric acid–ethanol and stated that it gave a purple coloration with the dicyanodiamide. According to Milks and Janes,[23] dicyanodiamide does not enter into a colour-producing reaction with 1,2-naphthoquinone-4-sulphonate in alkaline solution, although cyanamide could be detected through the orange-red colour it gave on heating.

(*b*) *Reactions of an Amino Group as part of the Amidino or Guanidino Group*

Dicyanodiamide yields a wine-red colour with α-naphthol–sodium hypochlorite in alkaline solution. This test for proteins containing the guanidino group is due to Sakaguchi.[34] He considered that an initial reaction stage leads to (4.7). Poller[35] studied the reaction later and

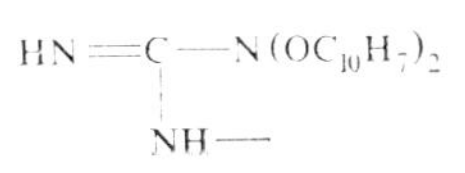

(4.7)

proposed a product in which only one naphthoxyl group was joined to the guanidino group (4.8).

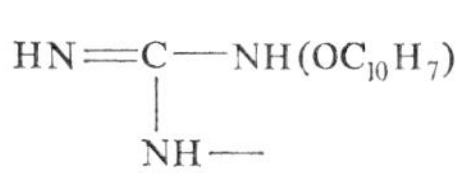

(4.8)

Knappe and Rohdewald[29] state than dicyanodiamide yields a purple colour with the reagent (using hypobromite) in TLC.

Another test for the guanidino group is due to Feigl and Costa Neto[36]. The sample is heated to about 250° (glycerol bath) and tested for evolution of ammonia with the Nessler reagent. Evidently two guanidino groups react to form the biguanidino group (4.9).

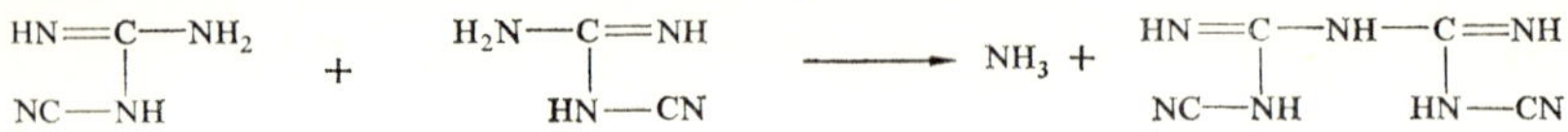

(4.9)

This test permits amounts down to 0·3 μg of dicyanodiamide to be detected.

(*c*) *Reactions in which Two Centres of the Amidino or Guanidino Group participate*

A colour reaction with biacetyl is described by Harden and Norris.[37] According to Feigl,[38] the test solution is heated to 100° with 0·1% aqueous biacetyl solution and a pinch of calcium oxide. A red-orange colour develops, sensitive to amounts of dicyanodiamide down to 10 μg. Probably reaction takes place with the enol form of the biacetyl (4.10).

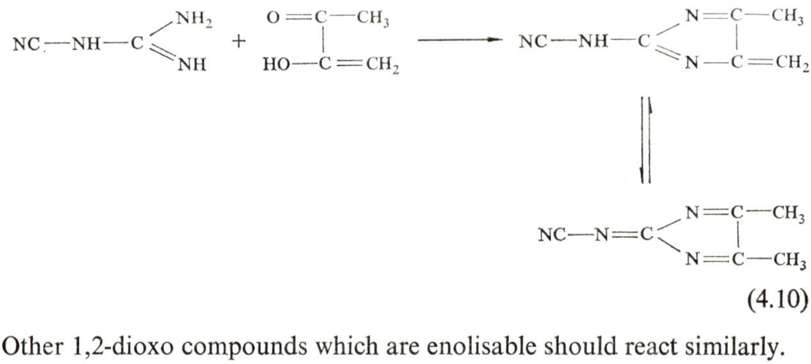

(4.10)

Other 1,2-dioxo compounds which are enolisable should react similarly.

A similar formation of a heterocyclic ring is postulated by Feigl and Yariv[39] as the first stage in a colour reaction with benzoin. Amidines yield imidazoles on heating with benzoin (4.11).

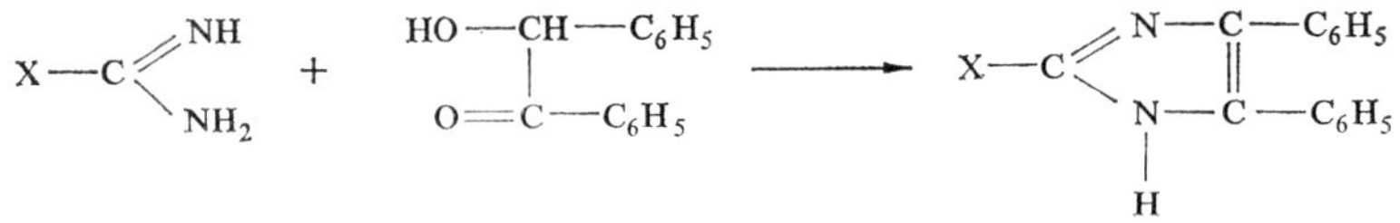

(4.11)

In the test for amidines, the tertiary nitrogen atom of the imidazole is then detected through the red–purple colour obtained on heating with 2% citric acid in acetic anhydride for 5–10 min at *ca.* 80°. Down to 5 μg dicyanodiamide can be detected in this way.

10. Cobalt in Vitamin B_{12} (Cyanocobalamin)

Strictly speaking this is a purely inorganic analytical problem and is therefore only touched on briefly here. Two types of method may be mentioned: (a) determination as cobalt(II) cation; (b) conversion to the dicyano complex containing $\mathrm{Co}\begin{smallmatrix}\diagup \mathrm{CN}\\ \diagdown \mathrm{CN}\end{smallmatrix}$, followed by its determination.

(a) Determination of Co^{2+}

This has been accomplished almost always by ashing followed by a standard inorganic procedure. These procedures include: polarography:[40] emission spectrography:[41, 42] colour reactions with nitroso compounds such as 1-nitroso-2-naphthol,[43] 2-nitroso-1-naphthol,[44, 45] nitroso R salt (1-nitrosonaphthalene-3,6-disulphonate);[46–49] titration with Pb^{2+} of the dithizone complex;[50] oxidation to Co(III) with hydrogen peroxide–sulphuric acid and its iodometric determination.[51] A preliminary separation of impurities such as free inorganic Co^{2+} or other vitamins, e.g. in multivitamin preparations, has sometimes been carried out; standard procedures were used, like extraction or ion exchange.

(b) Conversion to the Dicyano Complex

Most procedures here are based on the work of Rudkin and Taylor,[52] evidently the first to develop the method. The complex is formed by treatment with large excess of cyanide ion at pH 9·5–10 for several hours at room temperature. Spectrophotometric measurement at *ca.* 580 nm has usually followed. The complex has often been extracted to augment sensitivity and accuracy. For this purpose, solvents such as benzyl or butyl alcohols or phenol–chloroform have been employed and the extracted aqueous solution previously saturated with sodium or ammonium sulphate and its pH increased to 11–11·5; final re-extraction into water was usually carried out. The absorption maximum of the complex is at 578 nm but if differential spectrophotometry is used (comparison with the absorption of the normal mono-cyano compound), the difference in absorption is largest at 582 nm. Some investigators have measured the absorption at 367–368 nm.[53, 54] Preliminary purification of the cyanocobalamin before treatment with cyanide has occasionally been performed. References (55–65) give a selection of other publications based on this determination.

11. 5,6-Dimethylbenzimidazole in Vitamin B_{12}

Vitamin B_{12} gives 1 mole of 5,6-dimethylbenzimidazole on heating with conc. hydrochloric acid. Boxer and Rickards[66] developed a colorimetric and a fluorometric method for estimation of the vitamin, based on subsequent reactions of the imidazole, which they obtained by treating with 6 N hydrochloric acid for 18 hr at 150°. In both procedures, the imidazole is benzoylated with benzoyl chloride–alkali and the benzoyl derivative hydrolysed to 4,5-dimethyl-*o*-phenylenediamine with conc. sulphuric acid (4.12).

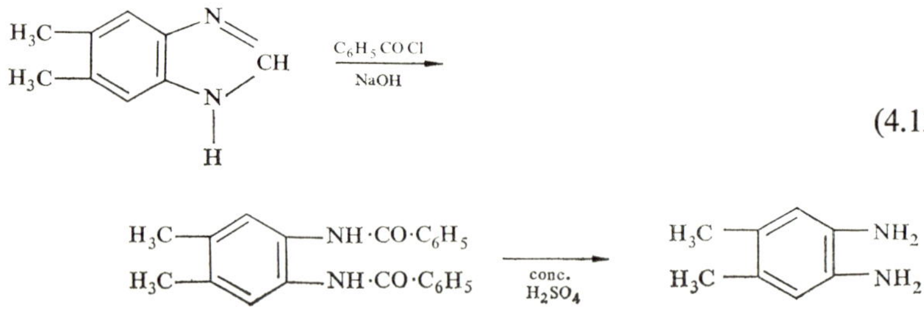

(4.12)

On partial neutralisation and treatment with aqueous acetylacetone for 3 min, the purple sulphate of 2,4,7,8-tetramethyl-1,5-benzodiazepine is yielded (4.13) on which absorbance measurements at 560 nm permit determination of amounts of vitamin B_{12} down to 10 μg. The fluorescent product is 6,7-dimethylalloxazine (4.14). It is formed in the sulphuric acid solution by reaction for 5 min at 100° with alloxan; the product is extracted with chloroform and then out of the chloroform solution with dilute potassium hydroxide solution. Fluorescence measurements are made on this alkaline solution, enabling as little as 10 ng of vitamin to be determined. The reaction schemes are given below:

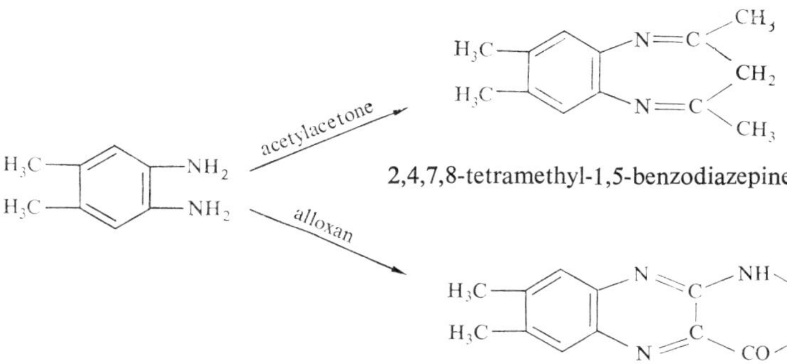

(as sulphate) (4.13)

2,4,7,8-tetramethyl-1,5-benzodiazepine

6,7-dimethylalloxazine

(4.14)

The methods of Fantes *et al.*[(67)] and of Heinrich[(68)] also depend on treatment with conc. hydrochloric acid. The former hydrolysed for several hours at 100° with 10 N acid, then shook the hydrolysate with n-octanol for 2–3 hr. An aliquot of the red alcohol layer was subsequently evaluated spectrophotometrically. Heinrich used 5 N acid for 1–2 hr and likewise esterified the "red acid" product with heptanol or octanol and measured light absorption at 552 nm.

References

1. TANG, H.-Y. and KUO, H.-F., *Jan Liao Hsueh Pao* **4**, 90 (1959); *Chem. Abs.* **55**, 3041 (1961).
2. IIDA, T., YOSHI, E., and KITATSUJI, E., *Anal. Chem.* **38**, 1224 (1966).
3. SUDBOROUGH, J. J. and THOMAS, J., *Proc. Chem. Soc.* **23**, 107 (1907).
4. LINSTEAD, R. P., *J. Chem. Soc.* 355 (1927).
5. LINSTEAD, R. P. and MAY, C. J., *J. Chem. Soc.* 2565 (1927).

6. HEIM, G., *Bull. Soc. Chim. Belge* **39**, 458 (1930).
7. OKHUMA, S., *J. Pharm. Soc. Japan* **75**, 1430 (1955); *Chem. Zbl.* **35**, 1705 (1964).
8. FLESZAR, B., *Chem. Anal.* (*Warsaw*) **9**, 223 (1964).
9. LUBATTI, O. F. and HARRISON, A., *J. Soc. Chem. Ind., London* **63**, 140 (1944).
10. SAHA, N. G., NANDI, U. S., and PALIT, S. R., *J. Chem. Soc.* 7, 12 (1958).
11. LADA, Z., *Chem. Anal.* (*Warsaw*) **4**, 375 (1959).
12. BOBROVA, M. I. and MATVEEVA, A. N., *Zh. Obshch. Khim.* **27**, 1137 (1957).
13. BOBROVA, M. I. and MATVEEVA-KUDASHEVA, A. N., *Zh. Obshch. Khim.* **28**, 2929 (1958).
14. DMITRIEVA, V. N. and BEZUGLYI, V. D., *Vysokomolekul. Soedin.* **4**, 1672 (1962).
15. MCBRIDE, W. R., HENRY, R. A., and SKOLNIK, S., *Anal. Chem.* **25**, 1042 (1953).
16. MAROS, L., MOLNAR-PERL, I., VAJDA, M., and SCHULEK, E., *Magy. Kem. Folyoirat* **69**, 123 (1963); *Anal. Chim. Acta* **28**, 179 (1963).
17. MAROS, L., SZAKACS-PINTER, M., and SCHULEK, E., *Anal. Chim. Acta* **25**, 546 (1961).
18. WAGNER, W. F. and KAUFFMAN, W. B., *Anal. Chem.* **25**, 538 (1953).
19. STREULI, C. A., *Anal. Chem.* **27**, 1827 (1955).
20. STREULI, C. A., *Anal. Chem.* **31**, 1652 (1959).
21. GARBUTT, J. T. and STRONG, G. M., *J. Agr. Food Chem.* **5**, 367 (1957).
22. HOFMANN, E. and WÜNSCH, A., *Naturwissenschaften* **45**, 338 (1958).
23. MILKS, J. E. and JANES, R. H., *Anal. Chem.* **28**, 846 (1956).
24. MAY, K., ROTHE, O., and MAY, L., *Melliand. Textilber.* **40**, 899 (1959).
25. TAKIMOTO, M. and KOEDA, K., *Kogyo Kagaku Zasshi* (*J. Chem. Soc. Japan, Ind. Chem. Sect.*) **63**, 797 (1960).
26. MILSTER, H. and MECKEL, L., *Textil-Rundschau* **16**, 593 (1961); **17**, 485 (1962).
27. WOGGON, H., KORN, O., and SPRANGER, D., *Pharmazie* **17**, 340 (1962).
28. ARDELT, H. W. and LANGE, P., *Z. Chem. Lpz.* **3**, 266 (1963).
29. KNAPPE, E. and ROHDEWALD, I., *Z. anal. Chem.* **223**, 174 (1966).
30. TAKIMOTO, M. and SAWADA, M., *J. Chem. Soc. Japan, Ind. Chem. Sect.* (*Kogyo Kagaku Zasshi*) **63**, 967 (1960).
31. LIST, P. H., *Z. Physiol. Chem.* **303**, 27 (1956).
32. KORN, O. and WOGGON, H., *Plaste Kautschuk* **11**, 278 (1964).
33. KORN, O. and WOGGON, H., *Nahrung* **8**, 351 (1964).
34. SAKAGUCHI, S., *J. Biochem. Japan* **5**, 25, 134, 140 (1925).
35. POLLER, K., *Chem. Ber.* **59**, 1927 (1926).
36. FEIGL, F. and COSTA NETO, C., *Mikrochim. Acta* 969 (1955).
37. HARDEN, A. and NORRIS, D., *J. Physiol.* **42**, 332 (1911).
38. FEIGL, F., *Spot Tests in Organic Analysis*, 7th English edn., Elsevier Pub. Co., p. 264 (1966).
39. FEIGL, F. and YARIV, S.; see FEIGL, F., *Spot Tests in Organic Analysis*, 7th English edn., Elsevier Pub. Co., p. 262 (1966).
40. ENDER, F. and STEEG, H., *Biochem. Z.* **321**, 426 (1951).
41. CARASSITI, V. and MIRONE, P., *Atti Accad. Sci. Ist. Bologna, Classe Sci. Fis. Rend. Ser.* **2**, 11 (1955); *Chem. Abs.* **50**, 7927 (1956).
42. MIRONE, P., *Ann. Chim.* (*Rome*) **47**, 526 (1957).
43. GAUDIANO, A., *Boll. Soc. Ital. Biol. Sper.* **29**, 471 (1953).
44. VARGAS, B. M., *Anales Fac. Farm. y Bioquim., Univ. Nacl. Mayor San Marcos* (*Lima*) **1**, 397 (1950).
45. VOROB'EVA, L. I., *Mikrobiologiya* **34**, 180 (1965); *Chem. Abs.* **62**, 12976 (1965).
46. MITRA, R. K., BOSE, P. C., RAY, G. K., and MUKERJI, B., *Indian J. Pharm.* **24**, 152 (1962).
47. MONNIER, D. and GHALIOUNGHI, Y., *Chimia* (*Switzerland*) **16**, 340 (1962).

48. BRUSTIER, V., CASTAIGNE, A., DE MONTETY, E., and ANSELEM, A., *Ann. Pharm. Franc.* **22**, 373 (1964).
49. MONNIER, D., *Arch. Sci.* (*Geneva*) **18**, 273 (1965).
50. EID, A. I., AMER, M. M., ABU-SHADY, H., and EL-MANGOURY, H., *J. Pharm. Sci. U. Arab Rep.* **4**, 157 (1963).
51. MENYHARTH, P., *Acta Chim. Acad. Sci. Hung.* **41**, 195 (1964).
52. RUDKIN, G. O. and TAYLOR, R. J., *Anal. Chem.* **24**, 1155 (1952).
53. SENSI, P. and LANCI, G. C., *Farmaco* (*Pavia*), *Ed. Prat.* **13**, 639 (1958).
54. COVELLO, M. and SCHETTINO, O., *Ann. Chim.* (*Rome*) **52**, 1135 (1962).
55. JANICKI, J., PAWELKIEWICZ, J., STAWICKI, S., and ZADROW, K., *Przemysl Chem.* **9**, 509 (1953); *Chem. Abs.* **51**, 2946 (1957).
56. VAN KLAVEREN, F. W., BANERJI, D., SHRIVASTAVA, P. C., and PATEL, S. A., *Current Sci.* (*India*) **22**, 142 (1953).
57. BANERJEE, D., *Indian J. Pharm.* **16**, 16 (1954).
58. KURMEIER, H., *Die Fischwirtschaft* **6**, 46 (1954); *Chem. Abs.* **48**, 7679 (1954).
59. VAN KLAVEREN, F. W. and SHRIVASTAVA, P. C., *Intern. Z. Vitaminforsch.* **25**, 139 (1954); *Chem. Abs.* **48**, 5955 (1954).
60. DE CARNERI, I., *Farmaco* (*Pavia*), *Ed. Sci.* **10**, 31 (1955).
61. OLLER, B. M., FERNANDEZ, N. G., and APARICIO DOMINGUEZ, L., *Arch. Inst. Farmacol. Exptl.* (*Madrid*) **8**, 55 (1956); *Chem. Abs.* **51**, 11436 (1957).
62. MARIANI, A. and VICARI, C., *Sci. Pharm.* **28** (No. 1), 41 (1960).
63. DOMINGUEZ, A., OLLER, G., and OLLER, M., *Galenica Acta* (*Madrid*) **14**, 157 (1961).
64. COVELLO, M. and SCHETTINO, O., *Farmaco* (*Pavia*), *Ed. Prat.* **19**, 38 (1964).
65. GSTIRNER, F. and BAVEJA, S. K., *Mitt. Deut. Pharm. Ges.* **35**, 29 (in *Arch. Pharm.* **298**, Heft 2, 1965).
66. BOXER, G. E. and RICKARDS, J. C., *Arch. Biochem.* **29**, 75 (1950).
67. FANTES, K. H., IRELAND, D. M., and GREEN, N., *Biochem. J.*, *Proc.* **46**, xxxiv–xxxv (May 1950).
68. HEINRICH, H. C., *Z. anal. Chem.* **135**, 251 (1952).

CHAPTER 5

DEGRADATION REACTIONS DURING WHICH THE CYANO GROUP REMAINS INTACT

Introduction

The degradation of compounds into smaller, more easily detectable or determinable products is a standard analytical principle. It is especially useful for compounds, such as polymers, which are often difficult to handle directly on account of their poor volatility or solubility, or low reactivity. The degradation may be pursued with or without an added reagent. In the present chapter, some procedures of this type are collected together. They involve reactions of cyano compounds in which the cyano group remains intact; in many of the procedures, it is this group, as HCN or cyanide ion, which takes part in the subsequent stage of detection or determination.

1. Pyrolysis without Added Reagent

A simple chemical example is due to Mano(1) who identified synthetic rubbers containing acrylonitrile by heating strongly and detecting the hydrocyanic acid evolved with a cupric acetate–benzidine hydrochloride–hydroquinone reagent (yielding a blue colour).

McConnaughey(2) also gives a test for hydrocyanic acid and for acrylonitrile in air or other gases, namely, the blue or blue-green colour given with an *o*-tolidine–anhydrous cupric sulphate–glycerol reagent; by using the reagent on an inert support, semi-quantitative estimation was possible by measuring the length of the coloured zone. Evidently the conditions of the test must be such that acrylonitrile suffers sufficient decomposition into hydrocyanic acid to yield a positive response with the reagent.

In recent years, the refinement of instruments has permitted the development of analytical techniques which are based on pyrolysis under standard conditions, followed by the application of a particular physical separation and/or evaluation method to the products. This provides a "fingerprint" of the original, pyrolysed compound. Under suitable circumstances, quantitative evaluation is often possible, based on a particular degradation product. Probably the most used "fingerprinting" techniques are infrared and mass spectra. Thus already in 1952, Zemany[(3)] applied this principle to polymers, studying the effect of various temperatures. Linear homopolymers yield the monomer as main product during pyrolysis at over 800°; mixtures are obtained at lower temperatures and also, of course, from mixed polymers. Zemany's examples evidently included artificial rubbers derived from acrylonitrile. Harms[(4)] in 1953 proposed a similar identification technique for natural and synthetic polymers. Pyrolysis at 350–750°, depending on the sample, was carried out; the products were condensed and submitted to infrared spectroscopy. Characteristic spectra were yielded. Amongst the examples were polymers based on acrylonitrile, such as Orlon, Dynol (copolymer with vinyl chloride) and Buna N (copolymer with butadiene), all of which showed the —C≡N stretching frequencies at 2200–2220 cm^{-1}. No attempt was made to identify any of the individual pyrolysis products.

A quantitative example is given by Bentley and Rappaport,[(5)] for the determination of acrylonitrile in Buna N phenolic resin blends. They heated 2 g samples for 5 min at a temperature rising to 550°, under 2 mm pressure, collecting the products in dry ice. After washing out with an acetone–chloroform mixture and evaporating the solvent, they recorded the infrared spectrum of the residue. The acrylonitrile content could be obtained semi-quantitatively from the peak height at 2216 cm^{-1}.

The above method, qualitative or quantitative, is not necessarily limited to polymers.

Chromatographic procedures of separation and subsequent "fingerprinting" may also be used after pyrolysis. In this connection one may mention the thermomicroseparation and application system (TAS) of Stahl[(6)] in which the sample is heated and the products deposited directly on to a thin layer; normal chromatographic development follows, yielding a chromatogram of separated components. It has been applied mainly to plant drugs and moderate temperatures are used, so that pyrolysis is negligible. Clearly, however, "low-temperature" pyrolysis may be carried out, yielding characteristic products of moderate molecular weight which are separable by thin-layer chromatography.

Mass spectrometry could be classified here since it depends on fragmentation into ionised particles which are then guided to form a spectrum according to their mass. It is, however, more convenient to deal with this later in the chapter on physical methods (Chapter 8).

2. Pyrolysis in Presence of Oxidising Agents

Several oxidative pyrolyses are described in the literature. Hydrocyanic acid is yielded and detected by standard methods. Thus Dezani[7] quotes a sensitive test for aliphatic and aromatic nitriles. The sample, plus an equal volume of hydrogen peroxide plus ferric chloride or sulphate are heated in a test-tube. Over the outlet is a strip impregnated with picric acid–sodium carbonate solution. The presence of a nitrile is shown by blue or, for very small amounts, by pink, red, or red-brown. Feigl and Amaral[8] describe a test in which the sample is heated with excess manganese dioxide to 130–140° for 1–3 min. Hydrocyanic acid is liberated and detected with the benzidine–cupric acetate reagent. Neither aromatic nitriles nor N-cyano compounds give the test but aliphatic nitriles in amounts ranging from 2·5 to 150 μg can be identified. Evidently HCN is evolved from the —CH_2CN group.

3. Pyrolysis in Presence of a Base

Feigl *et al.*[9] have detected aliphatic nitriles by heating to 250° with calcium carbonate–calcium oxide and identifying the hydrocyanic acid evolved with a benzidine–cupric acetate test paper held over the mouth of the ignition tube. The examples which they quote show that 2–50 μg amounts may be detected. Aromatic nitriles and other cyano compounds do not react. As Feigl suggests, HCN is presumably evolved from the —CH_2CN group.

4. Reductive Fission of *N*-cyano Compounds

In a test for the N-cyano group, Feigl and Gentil[10] use zinc and *ca.* 2 N hydrochloric acid and heat on the water-bath. The hydrocyanic acid evolved according to reaction (5.1), is detected by the blue colour with

$$=N-C\equiv N + H_2 + H^+ \longrightarrow =\overset{+}{N}H_2 + HCN \qquad (5.1)$$

benzidine–cupric acetate; from 80 μg (cyanamide) to *ca.* 200 μg (potassium cyanourea and dibenzylcyanamide) can be detected. The method is relatively insensitive because the hydrocyanic acid is partly reduced to methylamine. Nitriles with the C-cyano group do not give the test since they are reduced to C—CH_2NH_2.

Neubauer[11] used this reduction for quantitative determination of cyanamide in calcium cyanamide. After dissolving out dicyanodiamide and any urea with acetone, he treated the cyanamide in dilute acetic acid with Arnd alloy (Cu:Mg, 3:2). Subsequently, the solution was rendered alkaline with sodium hydroxide and the ammonia was distilled into standard acid which was back-titrated.

Feigl *et al.*[12] carried out the reduction differently for the identification of dicyanodiamide. They used a more concentrated hydrochloric acid (1:1, *ca.* 6 N) with the zinc, heating for 1–2 minutes at 100°. Methylamine and guanidine are thereby yielded (5.2).

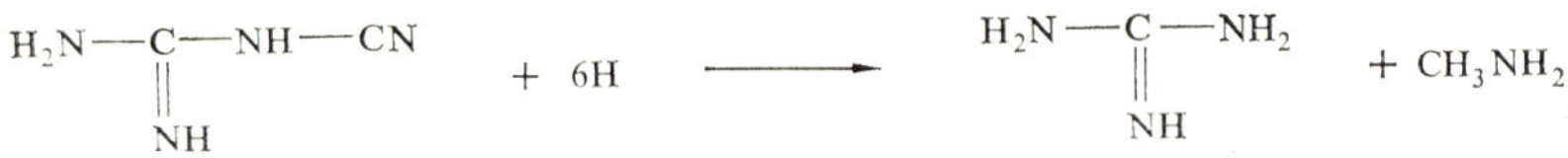

(5.2)

They then detected the guanidine through the red–violet colour with 1,2-naphthoquinone-4-sulphonate–alkali. Cyanamide does not interfere, since it yields ammonia and methylamine under these conditions.

5. Hydrolytic Fission of Cyanohydrins

Cyanohydrins are usually fairly easily broken down into hydrocyanic acid and the corresponding carbonyl compound by treatment with alkalies. This has been utilised analytically. Thus Ultée[13] determined cyanohydrins of ketones and of benzaldehyde (mandelonitrile) by decomposing with excess potassium hydroxide and then ultimately titrating the cyanide ion with 0·1 N silver nitrate. Berther *et al.*[14] determined cyanohydrins quantitatively by treating with a reagent containing nickel(II) sulphate in excess and ammonium hydroxide. The hydrocyanic acid yielded under the alkaline conditions forms $[Ni(CN)_4]^{(2-)}$. Unused $Ni^{(2+)}$ was then titrated with EDTA to murexide. Kraitsman and Chekhovskaya[15] determined lactonitrile in waste water from acrylonitrile manufacture likewise by decomposition into hydrocyanic acid in alkaline solution (pH 10) but their final stage was different. They used the reaction with sodium tetrathionate, yielding thiocyanate which was evaluated colorimetrically with Fe(III). Acrolein cyanohydrin in acrylonitrile was determined by Kuznetsova and Yamaleev[16] by reaction with sodium hydroxide–ammonium hydroxide–potassium iodide and then titrating with silver nitrate to the first turbidity; amounts of 0·1–3% could be estimated with an error of about 6%.

Berinzaghi's[17] determination of the nitrile group in acylated nitriles of aldonic acids, based on the Wohl method, can be included here. The sample in ethanol was treated for 24 hr at room temperature with ammoniacal silver nitrate; 1:1 nitric acid was then added, the precipitate of silver cyanide was filtered, washed with alcohol, dried at 90–100°, and determined gravimetrically. Deacylation and elimination of hydrocyanic acid takes place (5.3).

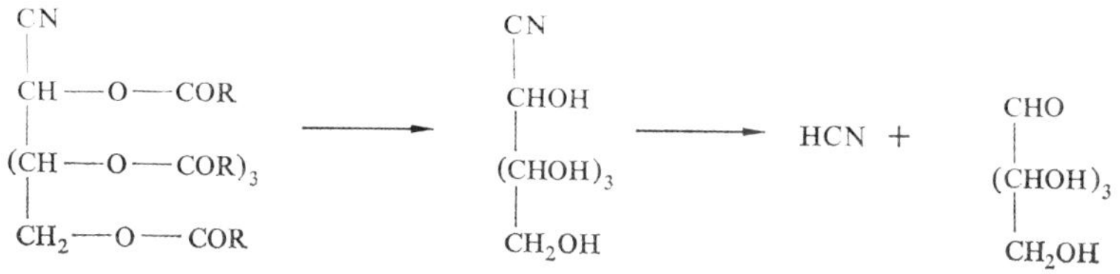

(5.3)

An interesting test which applies to cyanohydrins and is described by Feigl[18] can be appropriately mentioned here. It depends on the oxidation of *p*-phenylenediamine by hydrogen peroxide in acid or neutral solution to yield a dark product termed "Bandrowski's base" (5.4).

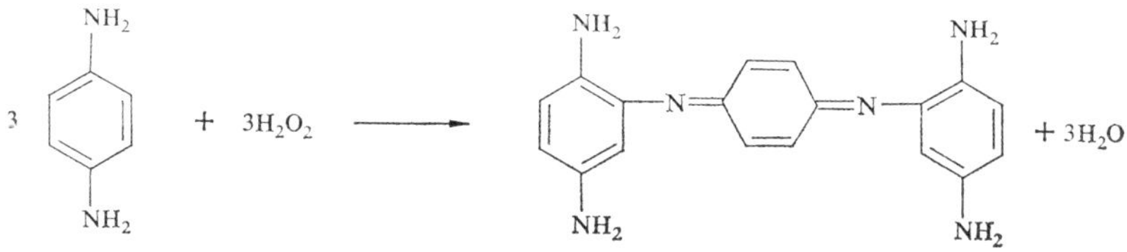

(5.4)

This reaction is catalysed by aldehydes and also evidently by aldehyde derivatives, which presumably exist in equilibrium with catalytically effective amounts of the corresponding aldehyde under the conditions used. Such derivatives include aldehyde ammonias, bisulphite compounds, and cyanohydrins. Thus down to 4 μg mandelonitrile can be detected through a yellow-brown and dark brown colour in acid solution and neutral solution respectively; with propionaldehyde cyanohydrin, it is rather less sensitive and yields a violet and a dark brown coloration in acid and neutral solution, respectively. Feigl's reagent consists of a drop of 2% alcoholic *p*-phenylenediamine solution, 2 drops 2 N acetic acid, and 2 drops 3% hydrogen peroxide; a drop of test solution is mixed with it. A blank is best carried out and the test should also be tried in the absence of the acetic acid; some aldehydes react more rapidly in acid solution and others in neutral solution.

6. Formation of Bromine Cyanide, BrCN

The reaction sequence (5.5)

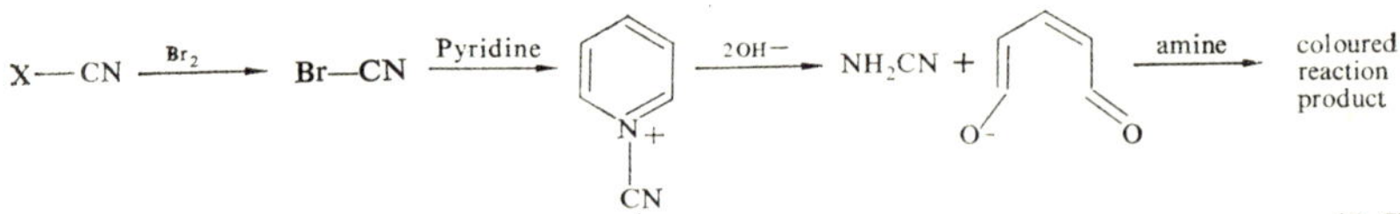

(5.5)

has been adapted to the quantitative colorimetric determination of cyano compounds. Thus Szewczuk[(19)] described a method for α-amino-nitriles. These were brominated with bromine–water–trichloroacetic acid for 1 hr at 37°, unreacted bromine was removed with arsenite, and then a pyridine–benzidine mixture was added. After 15 min, he measured the light absorption at 530 nm. A calibration curve was prepared from known amounts of potassium cyanide. Kanai and Hashimoto[(20)] applied the principle to the determination of acrylonitrile, brominating in light, destroying the unused bromine likewise with arsenite, and then adding also pyridine–benzidine. They measured the absorbance at 532 nm. The same authors later published the application of the method to the determination of acrylonitrile in biological materials.[(21)]

7. Elimination of the Cyano Group in the Analytical Methods for Ethyl Dimethylphosphoramidocyanidate (Tabun)

During the rush of interest in the so-called "nerve gases" from about 1955 to 1960, qualitative and quantitative colorimetric methods were developed which probably involved reactions of fission of the fluoride (Saran) or cyano (Tabun) groups on the phosphorus atom. Although this is by no means certain and although, also, the liberated cyanide ion plays no part in the subsequent analytical chemistry of the methods, it is convenient to classify the procedures here. Two types may be distinguished:

(a) Reaction with Peroxides under Alkaline Conditions

The probable series of reactions is shown in eqn. (5.6).

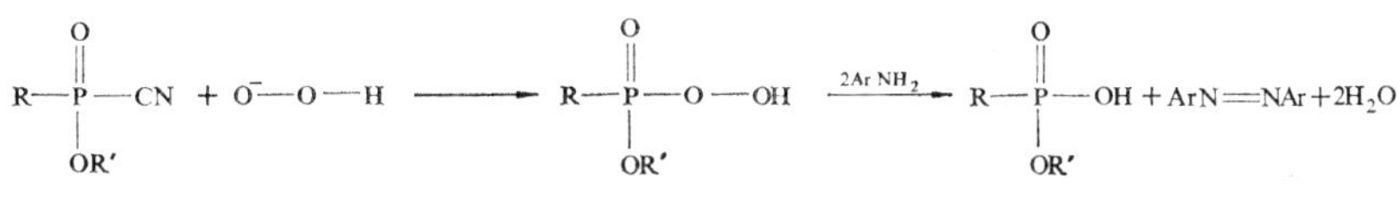

(5.6)

In the presence of an aromatic amine, the corresponding azo compound is yielded. The nerve gases (and other compounds such as acyl halides) function as oxygen carriers between peroxide and amine. The reaction scheme is simplified here, and it may be more complex. For example, when benzidine is used, the spectrum of the final solution differs from that of *p,p′*-diaminoazobenzene.

Marsh and Neale[22] used hydrogen peroxide and a dihydrogen phosphate–alkali hydroxide buffer, with *o*-dianisidine as the amino component; the colour was evaluated after 10 min. They studied the procedure in more detail later,[23] investigating the effect of pH, solvent, and rate of mixing of the reagents. Gehauf *et al.*[24] used sodium perborate (pH 10) and benzidine, allowing the mixture to stand for 20 min before measuring the absorbance; they stated that *o*-tolidine and *o*-dianisidine could also be used and that the absorption maxima were then at slightly greater wavelengths (440 and 455 nm, respectively). Koblin and Epstein[25] also used the reaction with *o*-tolidine for quantitative determination.

Gehauf and Goldenson[26] developed a more sensitive method for nerve gases, using alkaline perborate in acetone–water (1:1) and in the presence of indole. A green fluorescence was yielded, attaining a maximum after 30–60 sec. This was measured at 460–490 nm. Probably a similar oxidation occurs as above, giving indoxyl (5.7) or indigo white (5.8).

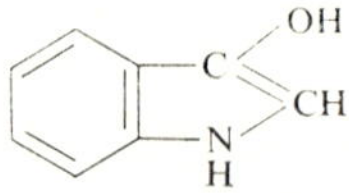

(5.7

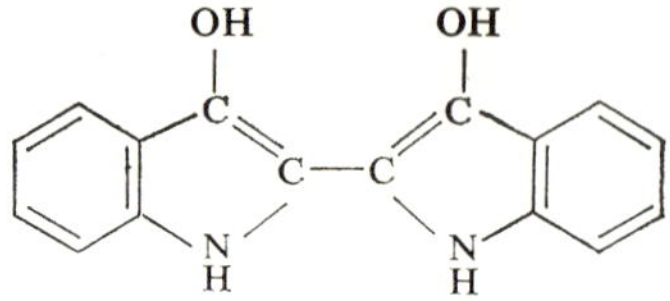

(or *trans*)

(5.8)

Both of these compounds show intense fluorescence. Hanker *et al.*[27] made use of this method.

Goldenson[28] worked out a chemiluminescence method for nerve gases, in which sodium perborate and luminol(5-amino-2,3-dihydro-1,4-phthalazinedione) were used, permitting detection of amounts down to 0·5 μg. Quantitative determination was also possible, since there was a linear relationship between concentration and luminosity. The classical luminescence reaction is with luminol–H_2O_2–$OH^{(-)}$/$Fe(CN)_6^{(3-)}$; the Fe–CN link is probably replaced here by P–CN (or P–F).

(*b*) *Reaction with Oximes*

Colour reactions with certain oximes, notably diisonitrosoacetone and 4,4′-bis(dialkylamino)benzophenone oxime, have been described as tests for nerve gases among other compounds. Three patents may be mentioned.[29–31] Sass *et al.*[32] developed a quantitative method, with diisonitrosoacetone at pH 8·4 (sodium bicarbonate or boric acid–sodium hydroxide); after 7 min, the absorbance was measured at 486 or 580 nm (magenta colour). Tabun could be determined in amounts down to 1 μg per 4 ml.

Little work appears to have been done on the reaction(s) involved. Sass *et al.*[32] postulate acylation of the oxime group with elimination of the halogen atom for the reaction with acetyl chloride. With Tabun, presumably the P–CN link would be broken analogously (5.9). The N–O link is then hydrolysed and another molecule of HCN is eliminated:

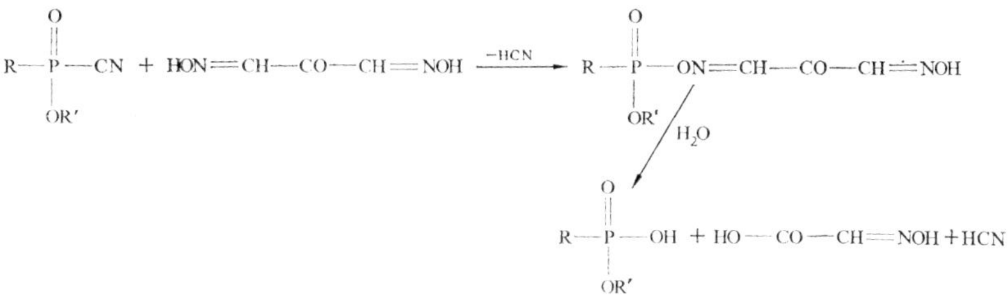

(5.9)

The isonitrosoacetic acid then forms coloured products, although no suggestion was made concerning their nature.

8. Elimination of the Cyano Group as Hydrocyanic Acid in Determination of Vitamin B_{12}

The elimination of hydrocyanic acid by adding a few drops of water and oxalic acid and heating serves as a test for vitamin B_{12}; the HCN is detected with the usual benzidine–Cu(II) reagent.[33] The elimination is the first stage in a standard method for determining vitamin B_{12}. Boxer and Rickards[34] suggested both reduction and photometric decomposition. They tested several reducing agents, hypophosphorus acid at 100° proving the best; others, such as ascorbic acid, formaldehyde, and glucose yielded volatile aldehydes which interfered. The reduction method suffers from the disadvantage that, under the conditions used, many biological materials yield some hydrocyanic acid. Photochemical decomposition has proved much more suitable. Wavelengths in the visible range are suitable, thereby eliminating any danger of photochemical side-reactions induced by ultraviolet radiation.

In the standard procedures, the hydrocyanic acid, yielded by irradiation for periods up to several hours, is swept out by a current of inert gas or allowed to diffuse out; it is then determined by a colorimetric procedure. One may mention: conversion with chloramine T to chlorine cyanide, then reacting this with pyridine–pyrazolone–bis(pyrazolone);[35–38] reaction with cupric sulphate–guaiac resin;[39] reaction with cupric sulphate–phenolphthalein–disodium hydrogen phosphate;[40] reaction with lithium picrate–phosphoric acid–pyridine.[41] Boxer and Rickards[34] freed the hydrocyanic acid from interfering contaminants by absorbing it in silver sulphate solution in very dilute acid in which it is retained as a stable complex and from which it is released by acidifying more strongly. It could then be collected in alkali and subjected to the colorimetric procedure.

9. Formation of Thiocyanic Acid by Reaction with Sulphur

Aliphatic and aromatic nitriles yield thiocyanic acid on heating with sulphur; this may be detected through filter paper moistened with acidified Fe(III) solution. Feigl *et al.*[(9)] were thus able to detect amounts of nitriles ranging from 1 to 20 μg; presumably it would apply equally well to N-cyano compounds, although these do not appear among the examples given. Sulphur can be replaced by thiosulphate.

Feigl suggests that the thiocyanic acid may result from the reaction (5.10) between hydrogen sulphide and thiocyanogen, two known products from the pyrolysis:

$$H_2S + (CNS)_2 \longrightarrow 2HCNS + S \qquad (5.10)$$

Aliphatic nitriles react faster than aromatic nitriles in yielding the thiocyanic acid; compounds containing the $-\overset{|}{C}=N-$ and $-\overset{|}{\underset{|}{C}}-N=N-$ groups also show a positive test.

References

1. Mano, E. B., *Revista Quim. Ind.* (*Rio de Janeiro*) **33**, 13 (1961).
2. McConnaughey, P. W., *U.S. Patent* 2,728,639 (27/12/59).
3. Zemany, P. D., *Anal. Chem.* **24**, 1709 (1952).
4. Harms, D. L., *Anal. Chem.* **25**, 1140 (1953).
5. Bentley, F. F. and Rappaport, G., *Anal. Chem.* **26**, 1980 (1954).
6. Stahl, E. and Fuchs, J., *Deutsche Apotheker-Z.* **108**, 1227 (1968).
7. Dezani, S., *Atti Accad. Sci. Torino* **52**, 826 (1917).
8. Feigl, F. and Amaral, J. R., *Spot Tests in Organic Analysis*, 7th English edn., Elsevier Pub. Co., p. 266 (1966).
9. Feigl, F., Gentil, V., and Jungreis, E., *Mikrochim. Acta* 47 (1959).
10. Feigl, F. and Gentil, V., *Mikrochim. Acta* 44 (1959).

11. NEUBAUER, H., *Angew. Chem.* **33**, 247 (1920).
12. FEIGL, F., GOLDSTEIN, D., and LIBERGOTT, E., *Chemist-Analyst* **53**, 37 (1964).
13. ULTÉE, A. J., *Rec. Trav. Chim.* **28**, 254 (1909).
14. BERTHER, C., KREIS, K., and BUCHMANN, O., *Z. anal. Chem.* **169**, 184 (1959).
15. KRAITSMAN, P. S. and CHEKHOVSKAYA, F. V., *Gig. i Sanit.* **30**, No. 6, 57 (1965); *Z. anal. Chem.* **230**, 65 (1967).
16. KUZNETSOVA, V. K. and YAMALEEV, I. YA., *Zavod. Lab.* **32**, 804 (1966).
17. BERINZAGHI, B., *Pubs. Inst. Invest. Microquim. Univ. Nacl. Litoral* (*Rosario, Argentine*) **17**, 50 (1953); *Anales Asoc. Quim. Argentina* **44**, 120 (1956); *Chem. Abs.* **48**, 11245 (1954) and **51**, 1777 (1957).
18. FEIGL, F. and FRANK, G., *Spot Tests in Organic Analysis*, 7th English edn., Elsevier Pub. Co., p. 198 (1966).
19. SZEWCZUK, A., *Chem. Anal.* (*Warsaw*) **4**, 971 (1959).
20. KANAI, R. and HASHIMOTO, K., *Bunseki Kagaku* (*Japan Analyst*) **12**, 754 (1963).
21. KANAI, R. and HASHIMOTO, K., *Ind. Health* (*Kawasaki, Japan*) **3**, 47 (1965); *Chem. Abs.* **65**, 14082 (1966).
22. MARSH, D. J. and NEALE, E., *Chem. Ind.* (*London*) 494 (1956).
23. MARSH, D. J. and NEALE, E., *J. Appl. Chem.* (*London*) **8**, 394 (1958).
24. GEHAUF, B., EPSTEIN, J., WILSON, G. B., WITTEN, B., SASS, S., BAUER, V. E., and RUEGGEBERG, W. H. C., *Anal. Chem.* **29**, 278 (1957).
25. KOBLIN, A. and EPSTEIN, J., *Armed Forces J.* **11** No. 5, 24 (1957).
26. GEHAUF, B. and GOLDENSON, J., *Anal. Chem.* **29**, 276 (1957).
27. HANKER, J. S., GAMSON, R. M., and KLAPPER, H., *Anal. Chem.* **29**, 879 (1957).
28. GOLDENSON, J., *Anal. Chem.* **29**, 877 (1957).
29. FISCHER, V. I., MILLER, J. I., SASS, S., and WITTEN, B., *U.S. Patent* 2,876,509 (6/1/59); *Chem. Abs.* **53**, 7865 (1959).
30. KRAMER, D. N., MORIN, R. D., and POIRIER, R. H., *U.S. Patent* 2,926,072 (23/2/60); *Chem. Abs.* **54**, 13502 (1960).
31. PFEIL, R. W., *U.S. Patent* 2,929,791 (22/3/60); *Chem. Abs.* **54**, 14510 (1960).
32. SASS, S., LUDEMANN, W. D., WITTEN, B., FISCHER, V., SISTI, A. J., and MILLER, J. I., *Anal. Chem.* **29**, 1346 (1957).
33. POHLOUDEK-FABINI, R. and BROCKELT, G., *Pharm. Zentralhalle* **96**, 503 (1957).
34. BOXER, G. E. and RICKARDS, J. C., *Arch. Biochem.* **30**, 382 (1951).
35. EPSTEIN, J., *Ind. Eng. Chem., Anal. Ed.* **19**, 272 (1947).
36. BOXER, G. E. and RICKARDS, J. C., *Arch. Biochem.* **30**, 372, 392 (1951); *Arch. Biochem. Biophys.* **39**, 281 (1952).
37. MONNIER, D., SABA, R., and GALIOUNGHI, Y., *Helv. Chim. Acta* **46**, 2558 (1963).
38. DOWD, N. E., KILLARD, A. M., PAZDERA, H. J., and FERRARI, A., *Ann. N.Y. Acad. Sci.* **130**, 558 (1965).
39. POHLOUDEK-FABINI, R. and BROCKELT, G., *Pharmazie* **14**, 253 (1959).
40. WIJMENGA, H. G. and HURENKAMP, B., *Chem. Weekblad* **47**, 217 (1951).
41. SEZERAT, A., *Ann. Pharm. Franc.* **22**, 159 (1964).

CHAPTER 6

DEGRADATION REACTIONS INVOLVING DESTRUCTION OF THE CYANO GROUP

VIGOROUS oxidation and reduction procedures are included here. Thus Kobayashi[1] proposed the use of detector tubes containing chromic acid–sulphuric acid on silica gel for determining acrylonitrile in air. The length of the green Cr(III) zone is measured for a definite aspirated volume of the air. The tube must be calibrated previously with known acrylonitrile concentrations. Amounts of 1–120 mg/l air can be determined. Takayama and Kadota[2] determined acrylonitrile in acrylonitrile-vinylpyridine polymers by treating with iodic acid–phosphoric acid at 220°; this yields nitrogen which can be measured in an azotometer. Pyridine is attacked only at higher temperatures (over 260°).

Thompson *et al.*[3] have suggested the identification of nitrogen-containing compounds through catalytic denitrogenation, followed by gas chromatographic detection of the products. They used 5% platinum on glass at 200°; their examples included benzonitrile which yielded cyclohexane. Beroza[4] also investigated catalytic reduction of a number of compound classes, detecting the products with a chromatograph equipped with a flame ionisation detector. His aim was structural elucidation rather than identification. On the palladium catalyst at 250°, benzonitrile yielded cyclohexane and methylcyclohexane as principal products; benzyl cyanide yielded methyl- and ethylcyclohexane.

Determinations of *N*-cyano compounds through conversion to ammonia by Kjeldahl digestion can be classified here. Léonard[5] determined cyanamide in this way.

References

1. KOBAYASHI, Y., *Yûki Gôsei Kagaku Kyôkai Shi* **14**, 673 (1956); *Chem. Abs.* **51**, 7240 (1957).
2. TAKAYAMA, Y. and KADOTA, S., *Kogyo Kagaku Zasshi* (*J. Chem. Soc. Japan, Ind. Chem. Sect.*) **62**, 140 (1959); *Chem. Abs.* **57**, 13972 (1962).

3. Thompson, C. J., Coleman, H. J., Ward, C. C., and Rall, H. T., *Anal. Chem.* **34**, 151 (1962).
4. Beroza, M., *Anal. Chem.* **34**, 1801 (1962).
5. Léonard, P., *Ing. Chimiste* **11**, 25 (1927).

CHAPTER 7

MISCELLANEOUS CHEMICAL METHODS

A FEW colour tests and some quantitative colorimetric determinations, the chemistry of which is unclear or as yet unknown, are given here. They are mostly used for particular cyano compounds.

Acetonitrile has been found by Morton and McKenney[1] to yield an intense red colour with trixenylcarbinol in glacial acetic acid. Some other compounds react similarly, e.g. nitromethane; water and dimethylformamide give a fleeting colour.

Barnard[2] stated that cyanamide reacts with haemin first to replace the chloride by cyanide and then further to yield a coloured product. He based a colour test for cyanamide in neutral or slightly alkaline solution on this. As reagent he used a solution of cetylpyridinium chloride in an isotonic phosphate buffer, saturated with haemin; a lavender colour within 15 min denoted a positive result and enabled as little as 1 part per 4000 of cyanamide to be detected.

Kunze[3] quotes a test for cyano groups, e.g. in polyacrylonitrile, by treating with diphenylamine in conc. sulphuric acid plus a drop of cold, saturated cupric sulphate solution; a blue colour is yielded, possibly following elimination of the hydrocyanic acid.

A quantitative colorimetric method for the determination of vitamin B_{12} in bacterial biomass and culture fluids is given by Velikoslavinskaya and co-workers.[4] It depends on the formation of an insoluble complex with Hg(II) in the presence of thiocyanate and chloride ions at pH 1·5. The precipitate is centrifuged, dissolved in excess ammonium thiocyanate at pH 8·0 and, following a purification procedure, the light absorbance is measured at 525 and 548 nm.

A recent rapid quantitative method for phthalonitrile is due to Hara[5] and enables amounts down to 2 μg to be determined. The sample is heated for 2·5 hr at 145° with hydroquinone–conc. sulphuric acid; water is then added and the solution extracted with benzene; the benzene solution is filtered and evaluated colorimetrically at 480 nm, or, better, the benzene solution is extracted with dilute sodium hydroxide and the absorbance of this alkaline solution measured at 595 nm.

Talsky[6] studied the colours yielded when anhydrous aluminium chloride is added to solutions of various compounds in dry chloroform (and, later, nitromethane and nitrobenzene). Aliphatic nitriles gave orange-yellow to orange-red colours; benzonitrile and phenylacetonitrile, red; and naphthonitriles and naphthylacetonitriles, greenish colours. He proposed the use of the colour test in group analysis.

References

1. Morton, A. A. and McKenney, L. F., *J. Am. Chem. Soc.* **61**, 2907 (1939).
2. Barnard, R. D., *J. Am. Pharm. Assoc.* **33**, 24 (1944).
3. Kunze, W., *Reyon, Zellwolle and Chemiefasern* 386 (1955); *Chem. Abs.* **52**, 9605 (1958).
4. Velikoslavinskaya, O. I., Grigor'eva, L. F., and Bukin, V. N., *Prikl. Biokhim. i Mikrobiol.* **1**, 155 (1965); *Chem. Abs.* **63**, 8716 (1965).
5. Hara, N., *Ind. Health (Kawasaki, Japan)* **4**, 30 (1966); *Chem. Abs.* **66**, 5542 (1967).
6. Talsky, G., *Z. anal. Chem.* **188**, 422 (1962); **191**, 191 (1963); **195**, 173 (1963); **201**, 203 (1964).

PART B

PHYSICAL METHODS

GENERAL INTRODUCTION

The application of physical methods for detection, identification, and quantitative determination has grown considerably in recent years. The following sub-groups may be distinguished conveniently, and they are discussed in the following chapters.

Chapter 8. Spectroscopic and spectrophotometric methods, including measurements in the infrared, ultraviolet, and visible regions; flame spectroscopy, mass spectrometry, nuclear magnetic resonance.

Chapter 9. Chromatographic methods, chiefly gas chromatography, which serve at the same time for separation. (The analytical chemistry of visualisation in column, paper, and thin-layer chromatography has been dealt with under relevant headings above.)

Chapter 10. Ion exchange.

Chapter 11. Polarography; although this could be regarded as a chemical method, it is convenient to accord it a special place amongst physical methods.

Chapter 12. Azeotropic distillation for separation.

Qualitative work is often concealed in publications on topics such as the separation and detection of representatives of numerous compound classes in industrial and naturally occurring mixtures (e.g. exhaust gases, petroleum fractions, tobacco smoke). It is impossible to scan every publication of this type on the offchance of a nitrile being present amongst the constituents identified. The information collected under "Physical Methods" is therefore largely quantitative, or is devoted to examples where cyano compounds have predominated in the sample(s) investigated.

CHAPTER 8

SPECTROSCOPIC AND SPECTROPHOTOMETRIC METHODS

1. Infrared

As long ago as 1948, Barnes *et al.*,[1] in an article on qualitative analysis, suggested that infrared absorption maxima be used as a means of identifying functional groups. The cyano stretching frequency between 2200 and 2400 cm^{-1} was considered especially useful for the identification of cyano compounds since it is in an infrared region free from fundamental vibrations other than triple bonds, or bonds involving deuterium. This means of detection has found widespread use and has become so self-evident that citation of specific examples appears to be superfluous. Two examples may be quoted in illustration: the work of Sokol *et al.*[2] on the identification of lower aliphatic nitriles in benzine (b.p. 60–150°) from carbonisation of brown coal (after preceding gas chromatographic separation); and the characterisation of higher straight-chain nitriles (C_{12}–C_{15}) by Iida and co-workers,[3] following separation stages with the help of urea adduct formation and column chromatography.

Table 8.1 summarises some information on quantitative determinations with the help of infrared data. Most of these concern acrylonitrile and its polymers and co-polymers; a smaller number deal with the estimation of other well-known cyano compounds such as ethylene cyanohydrin, dicyanodiamide, β,β'-dicyanodiethyl ether, and phthalonitriles.

The experimental techniques employed include the pressed disc method, prepared films, and solutions in various solvents. Acrylonitrile estimations have been based on absorbance measurements at 2230–2245 cm^{-1} (the stretching frequency of the —CN group, mentioned above). In determinations on rubber samples, the absorbance at this wave-number has usually been compared with that at another, notably the C–H stretch at 2970 cm^{-1}.

The information in Table 8.1 is given in chronological order of publication.

TABLE 8.1. DETERMINATIONS OF CYANO-COMPOUNDS WITH THE HELP OF INFRARED ABSORPTION ATTRIBUTED TO THIS FUNCTIONAL GROUP

Determination	Procedure	Wave number	Reference
Cyano groups in Buna N synthetic rubber	Sample extracted with various solvents, subsequently evaporated *in vacuo* yielding film on NaCl or KBr plates	2235	4
Acrylonitrile in polymers with butadiene (one example among many)	Concerned with development of new solid phase IR-lamination and impregnation techniques with mica, polyethylene, and AgCl	2245	5
Acrylonitrile from pyrolysis of rubber	Products collected in dry ice, washed out with acetone-chloroform, solution evaporated, and a pressed NaCl disc made from the residue	2230	6
Ethylene cyanohydrin and β,β'-oxydipropionitrile	Solution in chloroform	1060, 1130 and 965	7
Acrylonitrile in mixtures with styrene and butadiene	Solution in carbon disulphide	962	8
Acrylonitrile in mixtures with acrylic acid, ethylbenzene, methyl methacrylate, α-methylstyrene, and styrene	Solution in carbon disulphide	960	9
Polyacrylonitrile in coatings	Resin solution diluted with toluene	2230	10
Acrylonitrile in polymers with butadiene	Hot-pressed solid film	2920/2230	11
Dicyanodiamide	Pressed KCl disc	2170	12
Phthalonitrile mixtures	Pressed KBr disc	775 (*o*-) 810 (*m*-) 847 (*p*-)	13
Non-amines (including nitriles) in high mol. wt. fatty amines	Amines retained on acid form of Dowex 50W-X4; non-amines eluted with isopropanol, evaporated, and residue dissolved in chloroform	2240	14
Dicyanodiamide in acetoguanamine	Pressed KBr disc	2200	15

TABLE 8.1.—*cont.*

Determination	Procedure	Wave number	Reference
Small amounts of nitriles in long-chain fatty amides	Adsorbed on silica gel columns and eluted with $CHCl_3$. Evaporated and nitriles dissolved in tetrachloroethylene	2260	16
Analysis of reaction mixture from synthesis of amides from fatty acids	(Amides, amines, and small amounts of water do not interfere)	2250	17
Acetonitrile in isoprene, isoamylenes and their mixtures (for purity control of hydrocarbon fractions obtained by extractive distillation with the nitrile)	In solution in the hydrocarbons	2235	18
Nitrile groups in polyacrylonitrile	Pressed KBr disc	2240	19
Nitrile content of NBR–NR (nitrile-butadiene rubber–isoprene rubber, natural)		2260	20
α-(dimethoxymethyl)-β-methoxypropionitrile in mixtures with other (unsaturated) nitriles as intermediates in thiamine synthesis	Solution in carbon tetrachloride	2240–2260 (unsats. absorb at 2218–2232)	21
Dicyanodiamide in technical thiourea	Suspension in paraffin oil	2200	22
Phthalonitriles	Pressed KBr disc	769 (*o*-) 806 (*m*-) 844 (*p*-)	23

2. Ultraviolet and Visible

One of the standard methods for determining vitamin B_{12} depends on absorbance measurements in the 300–700 nm range; it has absorption maxima at *ca.* 278, 360 and 550 nm. The absorbances for 1 % solution in 1 cm cuvettes have been known for these wavelengths for over 20 years and have been utilised for determining concentrations of the vitamin; the two higher wavelengths have been particularly favoured (e.g. refs. 24–29). Comparison of the absorbances at two or more wavelengths (including that of minimum absorption, e.g. at 430 nm) has been employed also for controlling purity of samples (e.g. refs. 27, 30).

Spectrophotometric measurement has often been preceded by purification on ion exchangers (refs. 31–35), by paper or thin-layer chromatography (ref. 36) or by selective extraction such as between water and phenol–chloroform (ref. 28).

Bayer[37] drew attention to the change of absorbance in aqueous solution as a result of a photometric reaction in which the —CN group is replaced by —OH; he suggested that spectrophotometric measurements should be carried out in absolute alcohol or with aqueous solutions kept in the dark or at the isosbestic point (356 nm) between the cyanocobalamin and hydroxocobalamin.

Apart from these evaluations of vitamin B_{12}, measurements in the ultraviolet or visible spectrum have seldom been used for determination of nitriles. Table 8.2 contains some examples:

TABLE 8.2. DETERMINATIONS OF CYANO-COMPOUNDS WITH THE HELP OF ABSORBANCE MEASUREMENTS IN THE ULTRAVIOLET OR VISIBLE

Determination	Wavelength	Details	Reference
Acrylonitrile (in toxicity studies)	210 nm	On aqueous solutions	38
Dicyanodiamide in soil	215 nm	On aqueous extracts; urea, nitrate, guanidine, guanylurea and other decomposition products absorb elsewhere	39
Cyanamide–dicyanodiamide mixtures	225 nm	At pH 7 and 13, at which dicyanodiamide and cyanamide, respectively, absorb	40
Benzonitrile–benzamide mixtures	270, 274·8 and 277·2 nm	On methanol solutions; water and alcohols did not interfere	41
Acrylonitrile in presence of styrene	204 and 247 nm	Both absorb at 204, only styrene at 247 nm	42
Isomeric dihydroxy(1,2- and 1,4-)alkylated 3,5-dicyanopyridines	e.g. 367 and 337 nm	Example of 2,6-dimethyl-4-ethyl compounds	43 44
Terephthalonitrile	291·5 nm		45

3. Mass Spectrometry

Mass spectrometry has both qualitative and quantitative analytical aspects. Under definite conditions, certain modes of fragmentation are characteristic of certain structural features; this may be utilised to identify known compounds and to reveal structural details of new compounds. These are the procedures which are being increasingly used. As long ago as 1952, Van Meter and co-workers(46) used mass spectrometry for molecular weight determination in identification of benzonitrile, 2-methyl- and 3-methylbenzonitriles in shale oil naphtha fractions. Some other examples are: the work of Hartung and Jewell(47) on the identification of aromatic and cycloaromatic nitriles in petroleum products; of Merritt *et al.*(48) in identifying nitriles in the volatile components from ground coffee; and of Eustache *et al.*(49) for demonstrating impurities in acrylonitrile. Doubtless many other examples of this sort could be located and quoted but the difficulties in this connection have been stated already in the introductory remarks to "Physical Methods".

McLafferty(50) undertook a systematic study of the mass spectrometry of aliphatic nitriles; he considered that the spectra were suitable for identification and structure determination. Djerassi and co-workers,(51) however, drew attention to the difficulty, under standard conditions, of differentiating between the isobaric pairs CH_2 and N, and C_2H_2 and CN. One thus cannot always decide whether a given fragment contains the cyano group or consists of two species, one with and one without nitrogen.

The use of mass spectrometry in quantitative analysis of complex mixtures has been receding in recent years. This quantitative role is being taken over by other procedures, notably by gas chromatography. It has not been possible to find an example of quantitative evaluation of cyano compounds under standard conditions. Acetonitrile was, however, included in the compounds investigated by Varsel *et al.*(52) They used low-voltage mass spectrometry which often yields the molecular ion without fragmentation. The information about molecular weight thus obtained can be compared with data on functional groups furnished by higher-voltage mass spectrometry to permit identification. Proportionality was found also between concentration and molecular ion sensitivity, allowing quantitative determination to be carried out. Acetonitrile was in fact determined in a fifteen-component mixture by difference, since 1-butene and propene interfered too seriously in direct evaluation. No doubt, direct quantitative determination would have been possible on mixtures without these hydrocarbons or other similarly interfering components.

It is not intended to deal with structural elucidation in this monograph, but an example may be quoted. Griffin and Peterson[53] used mass spectrometry (amongst other techniques) first to show that a certain product was not a tetracyano- but a tricyano-compound, and then to distinguish between *cis*- and *trans*-tricyano compounds.

Since the first publication of Holmes and Morrell[54] in 1957, gas chromatography and mass spectrometry have frequently been coupled. Völlmin *et al.*[55] summarised the various ways of coupling, including arrangements with the gas chromatography detector and mass spectrometer in series or in parallel. Nitriles do not appear to figure in the examples of application but a large number of aliphatic nitriles from C_1 to C_6 have been found in cigarette smoke subjected to comprehensive analysis by this coupling technique.[56]

4. Flame Spectroscopy

Honma and Lothrop Smith[57] quote several nitrile examples in a flame spectroscopic method of detecting organic nitrogen. It was based on the cyanogen band at 3883 Å. Aqueous solutions of acetonitrile and alcoholic solutions of benzonitrile and chloroacetonitrile all yield relatively intense lines. A linear, quantitative relation was established also between percentage nitrogen and the log of the intensity ratio CN 3883 Å:CH 3890 Å (as internal standard), measured photographically. Ethanolic solutions of compounds were used, including nitriles such as acetonitrile, cetyl cyanide, α-tolunitrile, and malononitrile. The slopes of the curves of percentage nitrogen against log of the intensity ratio varied with the nitrile, being steepest for the more volatile nitriles. Down to 0·8 mg nitrogen in 3 ml solution could be detected.

5. Nuclear Magnetic Resonance

Structure elucidation, the principal field of application of NMR, is not dealt with here. An example may, however, be quoted of the application to quantitative determination of composition, namely of styrene–acrylonitrile copolymers. Černicki *et al.*[58] recorded the high resolution spectrum of solutions of the polymer in carbon disulphide, deuterated solvents, or liquid sulphur dioxide. It shows a field pattern at about 7 ppm, representing the ring protons of the styrene units and at *ca.* 1·5 ppm, representing the backbone protons of both the styrene and the acrylonitrile units. From the intensities of these two signals, the percent styrene (and hence acrylonitrile) could be calculated. In solvents such as acetone, the latter signal but not the former is screened from the styrene ring protons; comparison of the intensity with that from pure polystyrene also permitted evaluation of the mole percentage of styrene in the copolymer.

References

1. BARNES, R. B., GORE, R. C., STAFFORD, R. W., and WILLIAMS, V. Z., *Anal. Chem.* **20**, 402 (1948).
2. SOKOL, L., KVAPIL, Z., and KARAS, V., *Coll. Czech. Chem. Commun.* **26**, 2278 (1961).
3. IIDA, T., YOSHI, E., and KITATSUJI, E., *Anal. Chem.* **38**, 1224 (1966).
4. DINSMORE, H. L. and SMITH, D. C., *Anal. Chem.* **20**, 11 (1948).
5. SANDS, J. D. and TURNER, G. S., *Anal. Chem.* **24**, 791 (1952).
6. BENTLEY, F. F. and RAPPAPORT, G., *Anal. Chem.* **26**, 1980 (1954).
7. DUPRÉ, E. F., ARMSTRONG, A. C., KLEIN, E., and O'CONNOR, R. T., *Anal. Chem.* **27**, 1878 (1955).
8. KILEY, L. R., *Anal. Chem.* **27**, 1553 (1957).
9. SCHEDDEL, R. T., *Anal. Chem.* **30**, 1441 (1958).
10. ADAMS, M. L. and SWANN, M. H., *Anal. Chem.* **31**, 960 (1959); *Offic. Dig. Federation Paint & Varnish Prodn. Clubs* **30**, 646 (1958); (*Chem. Abs.* **53**, 20833 (1959)).
11. SMALL, R. M. B., *Anal. Chem.* **31**, 1742 (1959).
12. SUKHORUKHOV, B. I. and FINKEL'SHTEIN, A. I., *Izvest. Akad. Nauk SSSR, Ser. Fiz.* **23**, 1230 (1959); *Chem. Abs.* **54**, 6389 (1960); *Chem. Zbl.* **52**, 1712 (1964).
13. HADDEN, N. and HAMNER, W. F., *Anal. Chem.* **31**, 1052 (1959).
14. NELSON, J. P., PETERSON, L. E., and MILUN, A. J., *Anal. Chem.* **33**, 1882 (1961).
15. TAKEUCHI, T. and FURASAWA, M., *Kogyo Kagaku Zasshi* (*J. Chem. Soc. Japan, Ind. Chem. Sect.*) **67**, 2052 (1964); *Chem. Abs.* **62**, 12443 (1965).
16. BUSWELL, K. M. and LINK, W. E., *J. Am. Oil Chemists' Soc.* **41**, 717 (1964).
17. ZELENAYA, S. A., PANTELEI, T. I., and KOSTENKO, O. F., *Zavod. Lab.* **30**, 1077 (1964).
18. PASHCHENKO, N. M., SOROKINA, E. D., and BARANOVA, V. G., *Zavod. Lab.* **31**, 178 (1965).
19. DOERFFEL, K., *Wiss. Z. Tech. Hochsch. Chem., Leuna-Merseburg* **7**, 71 (1965).
20. TAKEUCHI, T. and MURASE, K., *Kogyo Kagaku Zasshi* (*J. Chem. Soc. Japan, Ind. Chem. Sect.*) **68**, 2505 (1965).
21. STERESCU, M., AFTALION, H., IONESCU, M., CILIANU, S., ROGOZEA, I., and IOAN, C., *Arch. Pharm.* **298**, 820 (1965).
22. SEIFFARTH, K., WOHLRABE, W., and ARDELT, H. W., *Z. anal. Chem.* **217**, 345 (1966).
23. SHMULYAKOVSKII, YA. E., ORANSKAYA, O. M., and BARANOVA, G. I., *Zh. Prikl. Spektrosk.* **6**, 681 (1967); *Chem. Abs.* **67**, 9082 (1967).
24. FORJAZ, P., *Anais Azevedos* (*Lisbon*) **1**, 163 (1949); *Chem. Abs.* **44**, 3675 (1950).

25. VARGAS, B. M., *Anales Fac. Farm. y Bioquim., Univ. Nacl. Mayor San Marcos (Lima)* **1**, 397 (1950); *Chem. Abs.* **47**, 4552 (1953).
26. MARSH, M. M. and KUZEL, N. R., *Anal. Chem.* **23**, 1773 (1951).
27. BACHER, F. A., BOLEY, A. E., and SHONK, C. E., *Anal. Chem.* **26**, 1146 (1954).
28. BUKIN, V. N., ARESHKINA, L. YA., and KUTSEVA, L. S., *Biokhimiya* **19**, 713 (1954); *Chem. Abs.* **49**, 6358 (1955).
29. CHEYMOL, J., *Ann. Pharm. Franc.* **14**, 589 (1956).
30. BRUENING, C. F., HALL, W. L., and KLINE, O. L., *J. Amer. Pharm. Assoc.* **47**, 15 (1958).
31. SAKOTA, N., IWAKI, M., YAMAMOTO, T., and KOSAKA, M., *Vitamins (Japan)* **9**, 302 (1955); *Chem. Abs.* **50**, 16033 (1956).
32. TAURO, C. S. and DIPACO, G. F., *Boll. Chim. Farm.* **98**, 460 (1959).
33. MARINI-SCOTTI, M., *Farmaco (Pavia), Ed. Prat.* **18**, 332 (1963).
34. MORA, G. A., *Quim. Ind. (Bilbao)* **12**, 141 (1965); *Chem. Abs.* **65**, 7907 (1966).
35. PETRANGELI, B., *Boll. Chim. Farm.* **105**, 770 (1966).
36. COVELLO, M. and SCHETTINO, O., *Farmaco (Pavia), Ed. Prat.* **20**, 58 (1965).
37. BAYER, J., *Chimia (Switzerland)* **15**, 555 (1961).
38. BRIEGER, H., RIEDERS, F., and HODES, W. A., *Arch. Ind. Hyg. Occupational Med.* **6**, 128 (1952); *Chem. Abs.* **46**, 11506 (1952).
39. PAWLIK, A., *Z. Pflanzenernahr. Dung. Bodenkunde* **89**, 181 (1960); *Chem. Abs.* **61**, 3692 (1964).
40. FINKEL'SHTEIN, A. I., SUKHORUKOV, B. I., KORNIENKO, T. M., and MUSHKIN, YU. I., *Materiali Tret'ego Ural'sk. Soveshch. po Spektroskopie, Inst. Fiz. Metal., Akad. Nauk SSSR, Komis. po Spektroskopie, Sverdlovsk*, 168 (1960); *Chem. Abs.* **58**, 9633 (1963).
41. ASTLE, M. J. and PIERCE, J. B., *Anal. Chem.* **32**, 1322 (1960).
42. BIRR, K. H. and ZIEGER, G., *Z. anal. Chem.* **196**, 351 (1963).
43. KUTHAN, J., JANEČKOVÁ, E., and HAVEL, M., *Coll. Czech. Chem. Commun.* **29**, 143 (1964).
44. JANEČKOVÁ, E. and KUTHAN, J., *Coll. Czech. Chem. Commun.* **30**, 1495 (1964).
45. MAKHTIEV, S. D., SALIMOV, M. A., SHARIFOVA, S. M., AGAEVA, E. A., and BABAEVA, N. L., *Dokl. Akad. Nauk Azerb. SSR* **23**, 22 (1967); *Chem. Abs.* **68**, 871 (1968).
46. VAN METER, R. A., BAILEY, C. W., SMITH, J. R., MOORE, R. T., ALLBRIGHT, C., JACOBSON, I. A., JR., HYLTON, V. M., and BALL, J. S., *Anal. Chem.* **24**, 1758 (1952).
47. HARTUNG, G. K. and JEWELL, D. M., *Anal. Chim. Acta* **27**, 219 (1962).
48. MERRITT, C., BAZINET, M. L., SULLIVAN, J. H., and ROBERTSON, D. H., *J. Agr. Food Chem.* **11**, 152 (1963).
49. EUSTACHE, H., GUILLEMIN, C. L., and AURICOURT, F., *Bull. Soc. Chim. France* 1386 (1965).
50. MCLAFFERTY, F. W., *Anal. Chem.* **34**, 26 (1962).
51. BEUGELMANS, R., WILLIAMS, D. H., BUDZIKIEWICZ, H., and DJERASSI, C., *J. Am. Chem. Soc.* **86**, 1386 (1964).
52. VARSEL, C. J., MORRELL, F. A., RESNIK, F. E., and POWELL, W. A., *Anal. Chem.* **32**, 182 (1960).
53. GRIFFIN, G. W. and PETERSON, L. I., *J. Org. Chem.* **28**, 3219 (1963).
54. HOLMES, J. C. and MORRELL, F. A., *Appl. Spectroscopy* **11**, 86 (1957).
55. VÖLLMIN, J. A., SIMON, W., and KAISER, R., *Z. anal. Chem.* **229**, 1 (1967).
56. VÖLLMIN, J. A., OMURA, I., SEIBL, J., GROB, K., and SIMON, W., *Helv. Chim. Acta* **49**, 1768 (1966).
57. HONMA, M., and LOTHROP SMITH, C., *Anal. Chem.* **26**, 458 (1954).
58. ČERNICKI, B. K., MÜHL, J. V., JANOVIĆ, Z. J., and SLIEPČEVIĆ, Z. K., *Anal. Chem.* **40**, 606 (1968).

CHAPTER 9

CHROMATOGRAPHIC METHODS

CHROMATOGRAPHIC methods have been used directly for separation and identification and also for the identification of components separated by other means. Many studies of mixtures of several compound classes have been undertaken and the inclusion occasionally of a nitrile in these cannot always be easily ascertained. This problem was mentioned above in the introductory words to Physical Methods; it is encountered most widely with the chromatographic methods, especially gas chromatography.

1. Gas Chromatography

Here, too, most problems have concerned acrylonitrile—the determination of its purity; as a residual monomer; as a product of reactions such as oxidative ammonolysis of propene and butenes. Acetonitrile has occasionally been determined in mixtures such as technical acrylonitrile or from oxidative ammonolyses also.

No particular liquid impregnation appears to have received special preference. Those employed include silicone greases; polyalkylene glycols; esters and polyesters; and higher nitriles such as β,β'-dicyanodiethyl sulphide. Likewise, no particular carrier gas nor detector type has been favoured.

Table 9.1 contains some published examples.

TABLE 9.1. GAS CHROMATOGRAPHIC IDENTIFICATION AND DETERMINATION OF CYANO COMPOUNDS

Compound(s)	Column and other details	Reference
Homologous series of n-nitriles (C_8–C_{20}, even numbers)	Carbowax 4000 monostearate on 30–60 mesh C-22 firebrick. 220–235°. Helium carrier gas	1
Acrylonitrile, methacrylonitrile, acetonitrile, propionitrile	(i) Carbowax 400 on Chromosorb W, 30–60 mesh, at 70°; (ii) 15% Craig polyester succinate on the same support, at 100°. Helium carrier gas. Unsaturated nitriles not separated from one another in (i)	2
Identification of many compounds, including lower aliphatic nitriles, also unsaturated	Done on a benzine sample from carbonisation of brown coal (b.p. 60–150°) and followed by infrared analysis	3
Analysis of high mol. wt. fatty acids and derivatives, including C_7–C_{18}; nitriles (from synthetic fatty acids, sperm oil fatty acids and sunflower oil)	Apiezon L on kieselguhr, at 276° (saturated and unsaturated nitriles separated at 240°). Hydrogen carrier gas. Thermal conductivity detector	4
Residual unreacted monomers (e.g. acrylonitrile) in aqueous emulsions of copolymers	10% stearamidopropyldimethyl-β-hydroxyethylammonium nitrate on Chromosorb W, at 100°. Helium carrier gas. Hydrogen flame detector	5
Identification of benzyl cyanide among many esters of phenylacetic and malonic esters	Apiezon L at 160–220° and polyethylene glycol at 220°	6
Analysis of aqueous solution of technical acrylonitrile (including HCN, CH_3CN, H_2O and acrolein); also of a condensate containing the same components (without water)	(i) Triethylene glycol on 600 grade firebrick of 0·25–0·50 mm particle size for first problem; (ii) β,β′-dicyanodiethyl sulphide for second	7
Aromatic and cycloaromatic nitriles in a hydrogenated furnace oil, after preliminary partial separation through $FeCl_3$- and $ZnCl_2$-complexes		8
Lower aliphatic nitriles in dilute acid solution (HCl); (saturated with KCl and dried extract with dichlorobenzene used for injection)	Diethylene glycol polyester adipate (LAC-2-R 466) + 2% phosphoric acid on Chromosorb W (30–60 mesh); 70° for mononitriles, 220° for dinitriles;	9

TABLE 9.1.—*cont.*

Compound(s)	Column and other details	Reference
	programmed from 70 to 220° at 10° per min for mixtures. Elution order of: acrylo-, propio-, butyro-(*o*-dichlorobenzene), succino-, adiponitrile	
Residual monomer in polymer emulsions (worked out for ethyl acrylate but tried also for a mixture with acrylonitrile). Toluene and hydroquinone added and partly distilled rapidly; organic layer of distillate dried and injected	30% Silicone stopcock grease on 30–60 mesh Celite 545, at 87°. Thermal conductivity detector. Helium carrier gas	10
Traces of acetonitrile in acrylonitrile	Various stationary phases tried—best was β,β'-dicyanodiethyl sulphide (adipates and phthalates also tried). Flame ionisation detector. Relative ±20% error for 0·01% acetonitrile	11
Separation of benzonitrile, nicotinic acid nitrile, pyridine and quinoline	Polyethylene glycol adipate on diatomite, at 180°. Hydrogen carrier gas. Micro flame detector	12
Residual volatile monomers, including acrylonitrile, in styrene-based polymers; solution or dispersion in dimethylformamide (+ toluene as internal standard) injected	Two columns in series: (i) 20% Tween 81; (ii) 10% Resoflex 446, on 30–60 mesh Chromosorb W. Nitrogen carrier gas. Both columns at 120°. Hydrogen flame detector	13
Impurities in acrylonitrile (acetonitrile, acetaldehyde, acetone, acrolein, salicylic acid)	Studied β,β'-dicyanodiethyl sulphide and oxide on brick carriers at various temperatures and rates of flow. Best was a 50:50 combination of 20% amounts of each, at 70–80°. Helium carrier gas	14
Aceto- and acrylonitriles in oxidation products of allylamine	10% Glycerol on column. Thermal conductivity detector	15
Cyanophenols in higher boiling phenols	Diethylene glycol adipate polyester +2% phosphoric acid on glass beads, at 180–200°; also polyethylene glycol monostearate on the same support	16

TABLE 9.1.—*cont.*

Compound(s)	Column and other details	Reference
Benzonitrile (also thiocyanate and isothiocyanate) in green plants; steam distilled and distillate ether extracted; extract injected	8% Butanediol succinate polyester on 80–100 mesh Chromosorb W, 190°. Nitrogen carrier gas. Flame ionisation detector. Also Apiezon L + Na capronate on Chromosorb P, 60–80 mesh, 200°; and 20% polypropylene glycol, 190°, with argon tetrode detector. Anethole as internal standard	17
Fumigants, including acrylonitrile	10% SE 30 on Dialoport S (60–80 mesh at 110°). Thermal conductivity detector, helium gas	18
Impurities in acrylonitrile (in amounts down to 1–10 ppm); acetonitrile included	20% Diethylene glycol succinate on Chromosorb P, 60–80 mesh, at 100°. Thermal conductivity or flame ionisation detectors; also coupled with mass spectrometry	19
Determination of the herbicide 2,6-dichlorobenzonitrile	High vacuum silicone grease DC-550 with Emulsogen WC 32, at 180°. Helium carrier gas	20
Determination of phenolic pesticides and residues, including iodoxynil and bromoxynil(3,5-diiodo-4-hydroxybenzonitrile and its bromo-analogue)	Dow–Corning high vacuum silicone grease on 80–100 mesh, acid-washed Chromosorb W, at 200°. Nitrogen carrier gas	21
Products from oxidative ammonolysis of propene (acetonitrile, HCN, acrolein, acetaldehyde)	Succinodinitrile on calcined INZ-600 brick	22
Aqueous solutions of acrylonitrile, dimethylformamide and various unsaturated esters	Polyethylene glycol 3000 or 4000 + dioctyl phthalate on polytetrafluoroethylene or stermachol, 80–90°	23
Separation of products from oxidative ammonolysis of isobutylene (methacrylonitrile, HCN, acetone, acrolein, acetonitrile, acrylonitrile, methacrolein)	Two-stage column: (i) 20% polyethylene glycol adipate; (ii) 20% β,β'-dicyanodiethyl sulphide, 60°. Helium or hydrogen carrier gas	24
Acrylonitrile content of NBR (nitrile–butadiene rubber) and NBR mixed with other polymers	Pyrolysis, then gas chromatography with a thermal conductivity detector	25
Dichlorobenil (2,6-dichlorobenzonitrile) in crop, soil and water samples (down to 0·005 μg/ml detectable)	10% silicone oil or 2% esters on Celite (100–120 mesh) at 100–163°. Nitrogen carrier gas. Electron capture detector	26

TABLE 9.1.—*cont.*

Compound(s)	Column and other details	Reference
Dichlorobenil in agricultural crops, fish, soil, and water	Electron capture detector	27
Straight-chain C_{12}–C_{15} nitriles in shale oil distillate, after separation through urea adducts and column chromatography	Identified by GC on a column of 2% SE-30 on silanised Chromosorb W. Temperature programme of 2° per minute. Hydrogen flame detector	28
Acrylonitrile and other impurities (such as ether and ethyl acetate) in ethyl acrylate	Triethylene glycol dibenzoate. Flame ionisation detector	29
Nitrilotriacetonitrile, iminodiacetonitrile (solution in aqueous acetone)	2% Versamide 900. Temperature programmed from 100 to 280° at 4° per minute	30
Reaction products from hydrogenation of adiponitrile (acetonitrile, hexamethyleneimine, hexamethylenediamine, ε-aminocapronitrile, adiponitrile)	Silicone elastomer E-301 on kieselguhr, treated with 4% KOH (146·5 cm), followed by 30% polyethylene glycol on the same support (3·5 cm) 155°. Helium carrier gas	31
Analysis of crude acrylonitrile from liquefied petroleum gases (HCN, aceto- and propionitrile also present)	16% Carbowax 20 M + 50% Kel F + 10% poly(*m*-phenyl ether) + 5% SE-30 silicone on acid-washed, 80–100 mesh Chromosorb W, all in a stainless steel tube	32
Traces of acetonitrile in acrylonitrile, plus water (from oxidative ammination of propene)	Study of columns. Complete separation of nitriles with mixture of 10% bentone 34 and 10% polyethylene glycol (PEG) 200 on Chromosorb P (60 80 mesh). 70°. Hydrogen carrier gas	33
Crotononitrile isomers and allyl cyanide	Polyethylene glycol 4000 + 6·5% silver nitrate on 80–100 mesh Celite 545, at 57°. Nitrogen, hydrogen, or air as carrier gas	34

2. Other Chromatographic Methods, Principally PC and TLC

Chromatography, especially paper and thin-layer techniques, has been employed for separating cyanocobalamin from other materials, such as other vitamins and factors and notably from hydroxocobalamin in more recent work. Separation has often been followed by quantitative spectrophotometric evaluation, based on absorbance measurements at one of the maxima such as 550 or 360 nm. A selection of chromatographic separations of this type is given in Table 9.2 below, together with references to the application, evidently relatively seldom, of paper and thin-layer chromatography to other cyano compounds. No special details of the visualisation and/or quantitative evaluation has been given since the methods used are mentioned elsewhere in the monograph.

TABLE 9.2. OTHER CHROMATOGRAPHIC SEPARATIONS OF CYANO COMPOUNDS

Compound(s)	Chromatographic details	Reference
Cyanocobalamin	PC; detected by its own red colour. Also electrophoresis, followed by quantitative determination through Co emission spectrometry	35
Vitamins, including B_{12}	PC, two-dimensional with buffered (Na-citrate–KH_2PO_4) water-saturated phenol and then with n-butanol–propionic acid–water. Vitamin B_{12} detected through its own colour	36
Vitamins, including B_{12}	TLC on silica gel; with acetic acid–acetone–methanol–benzene (5 + 5 + 20 + 70), B_{12} remains at the start and with water has hRf of *ca*.22	37
Non-cyclic cyanamide derivatives, e.g. cyanamide and dicyanodiamide	PC, using butanol–ethanol–water (4 + 1 + 2) and butanol–acetic acid–pyridine–water (4 + 1 + 1 + 2). Visualised with nitroprusside–ferricyanide–alkali reagent	38
Cyanamide	PC. Detected as Ag salt and quantitatively determined coulometrically after cutting out the spots	39
Dicyanodiamide from phenol–urea–dicyanodiamide resins	PC after hydrolysis. Visualised with nitroprusside–ferricyanide–alkali	40
C_{12}–C_{18} nitriles in industrially used lipids	TLC on silica, using one of three solvents: upper layer of benzene—N NH_4OH (10 + 1); $CHCl_3$, saturated with N NH_4OH–methanol (97 + 3); and petrol ether (b.p. 60–70°)–benzene (95 + 5). Visualisation with universal agents, notably charring with chromic acid–sulphuric acid	41

TABLE 9.2.—*cont.*

Compound(s)	Chromatographic details	Reference
Vitamin B_{12} after treatment with excess $CN^{(-)}$, then extracted with butanol	PC. Spot eluted with water and absorbance measured at pH 9 at 367 and 580 nm	42
Cyanocobalamin, separated from hydroxo- and sulphito compounds	PC, descending technique for 18 hours with sec.-butanol, saturated with water. Eluted with KCN at pH 6 and absorbance measured at 550 nm	43
Vitamin B_{12} separated from Factor III (also E and B)	PC, ascending technique with lower phase of chloroform–phenol–butanol–water (30 + 5 + 12·5 + 50). Paper first run with solvent, water or 0·5% KCN	44
Separation of cyano- and hydroxocobalamin	Studied TLC in 20 different solvents on silica gel G, buffered in some cases. Good results with butanol–acetic acid–water–methanol (20 + 10 + 20 + 5) or (20 + 10 + 20 + 10) on silica gel, buffered with 0·066 M KH_2PO_4; and with butanol–acetic acid–0·066 KH_2PO_4–methanol (20 + 10 + 20 + 5) on silica gel. Following scraping from the layer, spectrophotometric evaluation was carried out at 361 and 548 nm(cyano-) and 351 and 527 nm(hydroxo-)	45
Separations of cyano- and hydroxocobalamin, factors A,B(cobinamide) and III and pseudo-vitamin B_{12}	Studied TLC on several adsorbents. Established best solvents with preliminary circular technique: chloroform–methanol–water (65 + 25 + 4) and isoamyl alcohol–acetic acid–water (90 + 5 + 5) on alumina G; this latter solvent on kieselguhr G; acetic acid–sec.–butanol, saturated with water (1 + 99) on P-cellulose; sec.-butanol–water (83 + 17) on DEAE-cellulose	46
Separation of *cis*- and *trans*-tricyano-cyclopropanes	Column chromatography on alumina, eluting with benzene, ethyl acetate, and methanol, in that order	47
Cyanocobalamin, separated from hydroxocobalamin, etc.	TLC on alumina G with acetic acid–water–methanol–chloroform–butanol (1 + 4·5 + 5 + 10 + 25) or on silica gel G with the same components but (9 + 11 + 5 + 10 + 25)	48
Vitamin B_{12} from orange juice	Florisil column; eluted at 10° successively with water–ammonium hydroxide (40 + 10), water, propanediol–water	49

TABLE 9.2.—*cont.*

Compound(s)	Chromatographic details	Reference
	(8 + 42), water, and water–HCl–acetone (20 + 10 + 30); last named elutes the vitamin, then determined at 530 nm	
Separations of cyano-, hydroxo-, and dicyano-cobalamins. Aqueous solution of vitamin B_{12} treated with KCN, solution saturated with $(NH_4)_2SO_4$ and extracted with butanol	Butanol solution submitted to TLC on silica gel G or alumina G, using 95% methanol. Compared these fast TLC procedures, especially suitable for studying therapeutic preparations, with PC procedures	50
Small amounts of nitriles in long-chain fatty amides	Separated on a silica gel column, eluting with $CHCl_3$. Extract evaporated to dryness, residue dissolved in benzene and this solution subjected to TLC on silica gel G, developing with benzene which had been saturated with N NH_4 OH and dried briefly with Na_2SO_4. The spots, visualised in ultraviolet light (also visualised with iodine–Rhodamine B reagent), were transferred to paper and cut out; amount of nitrile was proportional to $\sqrt{}$area	51
Examples included cyanamide and dicyanodiamide, separated from urea and guanylurea hydrochloride or from guanidine–biguanide	"Centrifugal PC" using paper between two metal plates. Solvents for the cyano examples were n-butanol–ethanol–water (4 + 1 + 1) and n-butanol–acetic acid–pyridine–water (4 + 1 + 1 + 2); visualised with ferricyanide–nitroprusside–alkali reagent	52
Cobalamins	Separated on layers of silica gel–gypsum–NaCN, using descending development with water, saturated with sec.-butanol, at 22°; or sec.-butanol, saturated with water, at 50°. Plates ignited, then sprayed with β-nitroso-α-naphthol and Co determined at 367·5 and 240 nm	53
Vitamin B_{12}	PC (Whatman paper) or TLC (alumina or silica gel) by ascending chromatography; then densitometric evaluation	54
Cyano- and hydroxo-cobalamins and B_{12} coenzymes	TLC on CM-cellulose using lower layer of sec.-butanol–0·1 M acetate buffer of pH 3·5-methanol (4 + 12 + 1)	55
Vitamin B_{12}, separated from B_{12n} and factor V_{1n}	On Sephadex G-25	56

TABLE 9.2.—*cont.*

Compound(s)	Chromatographic details	Reference
Straight-chain C_{12}–C_{15} nitriles in a shale oil distillate; the nitriles and ketones isolated by urea adduct formation from distillate (pre-treated with alkali and acid to remove tar acids and bases)	Hydrocarbons separated from nitriles and ketones on a silica gel column. Ketones reduced to sec.-alcohols with $NaBH_4$ and separated from nitriles on a silica gel column with n-hexane–benzene (4 + 1). (Nitrile mixture then characterised by IR and hydrolysis to amides with H_2SO_4 and subsequently separated by GC)	28
Separation of cyano- and hydroxocobalamin	TLC on neutral alumina; best solvent system was isobutanol–isopropanol–water (6 + 4 + 5), plus ammonium hydroxide to bring to pH 8·5. Rf values of 0·46 and 0·30 respectively	57
Nitrogen derivatives of carbonic acid, including cyanamide and dicyanodiamide	TLC on cellulose, using methanol-3 N ammonium hydroxide (60 + 75); or on highly pure silica gel, with acetonitrile–petrol ether–carbon tetrachloride–tetrahydrofuran–water–formic acid (80 + 10 + 10 + 10 + 10 + 4). Visualised with various colour reagents (see pp. 54, 60)	58
Aliphatic dinitriles (C_3–C_8), separated from corresponding ammonium salts and amides and amines derived by hydrogenation	TLC on silica gel G layers, using chloroform (saturated with 10% sulphuric acid)-butanone-2 (or pentanone-2) (95 + 5); nitriles separated from one another by multiple development. Visualisation by hydrolysis using H_2O_2–H_2SO_4 and then spraying with *p*-nitrobenzene–diazonium salt, followed with NaOH, giving red spots	59

References

1. LINK, W. E., HICKMAN, H. M., and MORRISSETTE, R. A., *J. Am. Oil Chemists' Assoc.* **36**, 20 (1959).
2. LYSYJ, I., *Anal. Chem.* **32**, 771 (1960).
3. SOKOL, L., KVAPIL, Z., and KARAS, V., *Coll. Czech. Chem. Commun.* **26**, 2278 (1961).
4. VASILESCU, V., *Fette Seifen. Anstrichmittel*, **63**, 132 (1961).
5. SHAPRAS, P. and CLAVER, G. C., *Anal. Chem.* **34**, 433 (1962).
6. JANÁK, J., NOVÁK, J., and SULOVSKÝ, J., *Coll. Czech. Chem. Commun.* **27**, 2541 (1962).
7. BORODULINA, R. I., VERTEBNYI, P. YA., and REVEL'SKII, I. A., *Gaz. Khromatogr. Akad. Nauk SSSR, Tr. Vtoroi Vses. Konf. Moscow* 317 (1962); *Chem. Abs.* **62**, 5894 (1965).

8. Hartung, G. K. and Jewell, D. M., *Anal. Chim. Acta* **27**, 219 (1962).
9. Arad-Talmi, Y., Levy, M., and Vofsi, D., *J. Chromatog.* **10**, 417 (1963).
10. Tweet, O. and Miller, W. K., *Anal. Chem.* **35**, 852 (1963).
11. Borodulina, R. I., Revel'skii, I. A., and Shtylenko, A. D., *Plast. Massy* 49 (1964).
12. Chekmareva, I. B., Trubnikov, V. I., and Bereskin, W. G., *Zh. Anal. Khim.* **19**, 395 (1964).
13. Shapras, P. and Claver, G. C., *Anal. Chem.* **36**, 2282 (1964).
14. Sakodynskii, K. I., Khokhlova, L. A., Brazhnikov, V. V., and Sevryugova, N. N., *Gazov Khromatogr.* No. 1, 96 (1964); *Chem. Abs.* **67**, 5697 (1967).
15. Hsieh, H.-F. and Chang, T.Ch., *Chung Kuo K'o Hsueh Yuan Ying Yung Hua Hsueh Yen Chiu So Chi K'an* 68 (1964); *Chem. Abs.* **64**, 1355 (1966).
16. Lindsay Smith, J. R., Norman, R. O. C., and Radda, G. K., *J. Gas Chromatog.* **2**, 146 (1964).
17. Wahlroos, Ö. and Saarivirta, M., *Acta Chem. Scand.* **18**, 2191 (1964).
18. Berck, B., *J. Agr. Food Chem.* **13**, 373 (1965).
19. Eustache, H., Guillemin, C. L., and Auricourt, F., *Bull. Soc. Chim. France* 1386 (1965).
20. Kanazawa, J., *Bunseki Kagaku* (*Japan Analyst*) **14**, 720 (1965).
21. Gutenmann, W. H. and List, D. J., *J. Assoc. Offic. Agr. Chem.* **48**, 1173 (1965).
22. Nikolaeva, M. M. and Serebryakov, B. R., *Gaz. Khromatogr., Moscow* No. 3, 28 (1965); *Chem. Abs.* **66**, 9500 (1967).
23. Nestler, H. and Berger, W., *Chem. Tech.* (*Berlin*) **17**, 169 (1965).
24. Nikolaeva, N. M. and Fonkich, A. G., *Gazov. Khromatogr.* No. 3, 149 (1965); *Chem. Abs.* **68**, 4451 (1968).
25. Cole, H. M., Petterson, D. L., Sljaka, V. A., and Smith, D. S., *Rubber Chem. Technol.* **39**, 259 (1966).
26. Beynon, K. I., Davies, L., Elgar, K., and Wright, A. N., *J. Sci. Food Agr.* **17**, 151, 156 (1966).
27. Meulemans, K. J. and Upton, E. T., *J. Assoc. Off. Agric. Chem.* **49**, 976 (1966).
28. Iida, T., Yoshi, E., and Kitatsuji, E., *Anal. Chem.* **38**, 1224 (1966).
29. Lyutova, T. M. and Lazaris, A. Ya., *Zh. Anal. Khim.* **21**, 1146 (1966).
30. Weissert, N. H. and Coelho, R. A., *J. Gas Chromatog.* **5**, 160 (1967).
31. Arakelyan, V. G., Sarycheva, L. S., Bobyleva, L. I., Trofil'kina, V. P., and Evdakov, V. P., *Zh. Anal. Khim.* **22**, 618 (1967).
32. Li, Shih-Chang and Huang, Wu-Tong, *J. Chinese Chem. Soc.* (*Taipeh*) **14**, 108 (1967); *Chem. Abs.* **68**, 10721 (1968).
33. Dandoy, J., *J. Chromatog.* **32**, 184 (1968).
34. Mirzayanov, V. S. and Grechko, V. A., *Zh. Anal. Khim.* **23**, 109 (1968).
35. Carassiti, V. and Mirone, P., *Atti Accad. Sci. Ist., Bologna, Classe Sci. Fis. Rend. Ser.* **2**, 11 (1955); *Chem. Abs.* **50**, 7927 (1956).
36. Gadsden, E. L., Edwards, C. H., and Edwards, G. A., *Anal. Chem.* **32**, 1415 (1960).
37. Gänshirt, H. and Malzacher, A., *Naturwissenschaften* **47**, 279 (1960).
38. Takimoto, M. and Koeda, K., *J. Chem. Soc. Japan* (*Kogyo Kagaku Zasshi*) **63**, 797 (1960).
39. Yamada, T. and Sakai, Y., *Denki Kagaku* (*J. Electrochem. Soc. Japan*) **29**, 852 (1961).
40. Meckel, L. and Milster, H., *Textil-Rundschau* **16**, 593 (1961); **17**, 485 (1962).
41. Mangold, H. K. and Kammereck, R., *J. Am. Oil Chemists' Soc.* **39**, 201 (1962).
42. Covello, M. and Schettino, O., *Ann. Chim.* (*Rome*) **52**, 1135 (1962).

43. CARDINI, C., CAVINA, G., CINGOLANI, E., MARIANI, A., and VICARI, C., *Farmaco (Pavia), Ed. Prat.* **17**, 583 (1962).
44. BAYER, J., *J. Chromatog.* **8**, 123 (1962).
45. CIMA, L. and MANTOVAN, R., *Farmaco (Pavia), Ed. Prat.* **17**, 473 (1962).
46. HAYASHI, M. and KAMIKUBO, T., *J. Vitaminol (Kyoto)* **11**, 286 (1963).
47. GRIFFIN, G. W. and PETERSON, L. I., *J. Org. Chem.* **28**, 3219 (1963).
48. ONE, T., *Bitamin (Kyoto)* **30**, 280 (1964); *Chem. Abs.* **62**, 1957 (1965).
49. RAHANDRAHA, T., CHANEZ, M., and SAGOT-MASSON, M., *Ann. Pharm. Franc.* **22**, 663 (1964).
50. COVELLO, M. and SCHETTINO, O., *Farmaco (Pavia), Ed. Prat.* **19**, 38 (1964).
51. BUSWELL, K. M. and LINK, W. E., *J. Am. Oil Chemists' Soc.* **41**, 717 (1964).
52. LOWERY, J. A. and CASSIDY, J. E., *J. Chromatog.* **13**, 467 (1964).
53. VOROB'EVA, L. I., *Mikrobiologiya* **34**, 180 (1965).
54. COVELLO, M. and SCHETTINO, O., *Farmaco (Pavia), Ed. Prat.* **20**, 581 (1965).
55. SASAKI, T., *J. Chromatog.* **24**, 452 (1966).
56. PEKEL, N. D. and BEREZOVSKII, V. M., *Med. Prom. SSSR* **20**, 21 (1966); *Chem. Abs.* **66**, 11049 (1967).
57. POPOVA, YA., POPOV, C., and ILIEVA, M., *J. Chromatog.* **24**, 263 (1966).
58. KNAPPE, E. and ROHDEWALD, I., *Z. anal. Chem.* **223**, 174 (1966).
59. EULENHOEFER, H. G., *J. Chromatog.* **36**, 198 (1968).

CHAPTER 10

ION EXCHANGE

THERE seem to be no publications about the use of ion exchangers for preliminary purification and/or separation of nitriles or other cyano compounds, except of cyanocobalamin. Marsh and Kuzel[1] were evidently the first to free vitamin B_{12} from interfering compounds, such as other vitamins, using this technique. Both anionic and cationic exchangers have been used, the latter predominating slightly. The exchanger or exchangers employed have, of course, depended on the nature of the sample and problem and conditions of the determination. Table 10.1 contains some examples.

TABLE 10.1. SEPARATION OF VITAMIN B_{12} ON ION EXCHANGERS

Sample	Ion exchanger	Further details	Reference
Synthetic vitamin mixtures	Many tested and a combination proposed of anionic Amberlite IRA 400, regenerated with 10% NaOH below 1:1 mixture of the same and of cationic Amberlite IRC 120, regenerated with 2·5% or with 10% H_2SO_4	Final spectrophotometric evaluation at 550 nm	1
Multivitamin preparations	Strongly basic anionic ion exchangers; Amberlite IRA-410 best, IRA-400 also good	Final spectrophotometric evaluation of B_{12} at 550 nm (riboflavin interferes at 361 nm)	2
Vitamin B_{12} in liver injections; hydroxo- and other cobalamins converted to	Cationic Amberlite XE-97, treated with citrate buffer to bring to pH 4	Cyanocobalamin solution brought to pH4 with citrate buffer; contaminants eluted with HCl and then	3

TABLE 10.1.—*cont.*

Sample	Ion exchanger	Further details	Reference
cyano- by treatment with KCN at pH 7·5 for 3 hours		acetone; cyanocobalamin then eluted with dioxan–HCl, converted to the dicyano complex and evaluated at 578 nm	
Vitamin B_{12}	Adsorbed on Amberlite IRC 50 (weakly cationic) and eluted with 0·1 N HCl 75% acetone		4
Vitamin B_{12} in mixture with adenosine-5-monophosphate	Amberlite IR 410, pretreated with NaOH	Spectrophotometry at 260 nm	5
	Cyanocobalamin retained by various cationic exchangers (e.g. Dowex 50, Amberlite XE 69, Merck Austauscher IV), pretreated with NH_4Cl at a definite pH, yielding a particular $NH_4^{(+)}$–$H^{(+)}$ ratio in the resin		6
Separation and purification of vitamin B_{12}	Cationic exchange resin SDV 3 in $H^{(+)}$–form studied	Vitamin displaced by cations, thus appearing in the effluent	7
Polyvitamin preparations	Amberlite IRA 400 and others	Vitamin B_{12} then determined by conversion into the dicyano complex and spectrophotometry	8
Traces of vitamin B_{12} in polyvitamin preparations	Amberlite CG 50 (cationic exchanger)	Vitamin eluted with dioxan–HCl and ultimately evaluated by ashing and Co determination	9
Vitamin B_{12} in mixture with uridine-5-triphosphate in lyophilised preparations	Anionic Dowex 1-X8	Determined through absorbance at 361 nm	10

TABLE 10.1.—*cont.*

Sample	Ion exchanger	Further details	Reference
Separation of cyano- and hydroxo-cobalamins; quantitative evaluation of vitamin B_{12}	Numerous Amberlite papers pre-treated and tested under different conditions with water and dioxan–N HCl mixtures as eluents. Best quantitative results with cationic ion-exchange paper Amberlite WA-2 (Type Amberlite IRC 50) buffered at pH 4·6 by standing 1 hr in acetate buffer and drying overnight	Eluted with dioxan-N HCl–water (3 + 1 + 6); hydroxo- migrates only little, cyano- almost with the solvent front. For quantitative determination hydroxo-spot first converted to cyano- with KCN; then eluted with acetone (50%) containing 7·5% NaCl, and light absorbance finally measured at 361 nm	11
Cyano-, hydroxo-cobalamins, folic acid and nicotinamide	DEAE-cellulose, then CMC-cellulose	Absorbance of percolate measured at 361 nm	12
Cyanocobalamin in injection solutions	Slight modification of method of ref. (3)		13
Vitamin B_{12} in vitamin B complex solutions	Wofatit CP 300	Other vitamins eluted with water and 0·01 N HCl–water–acetone; final spectrophotometry at 361 nm	14
Vitamin B_{12} in concentrates and mixed feed supplements	Amberlite CG 50, treated with alkali	Eluted with dioxan–HCl and evaluated at 550 nm	15
Cyanocobalamin in syrups	Amberlite XE 97, treated with citrate buffer, pH 4, as in ref. (3)	Eluted with dioxan–HCl and determined spectrophotometrically	16
Separation of B_{12} from B_{12n} and factor V_{1n}	Sephadex G 25		17

References

1. MARSH, M. M. and KUZEL, N. R., *Anal. Chem.* **23**, 1773 (1951).
2. SAKOTA, N., IWAKI, M., YAMAMOTO, T., and KOSAKA, M., *Bitamin* (*Kyoto*) **9**, 302 (1955); *Chem. Abs.* **50**, 16033 (1956).

3. VAN MELLE, P. J., *J. Am. Pharm. Assoc.* **45**, 26 (1956).
4. KAMIKUBO, T. and TANAKE, T., *Bitamin* (*Kyoto*) **10**, 424 (1956); *Chem. Abs.* **51**, 18404 (1957).
5. OLIVARI, G., *Boll. Chim. Farm.* **97**, 263 (1958).
6. MENKE, K. H., *Naturwissenschaften* **45**, 263 (1958).
7. EL'KIN, G. E., KLIKH, S. F., and SAMSONOV, G. V., *Zh. Prikl. Khim.* **33**, 1397 (1960).
8. DOMINGUEZ, A., OLLER, G., and OLLER, M., *Galenica Acta* (*Madrid*) **14**, 157 (1961).
9. MONNIER, D. and GHALIOUNGHI, Y., *Chimia* (*Switzerland*) **16**, 340 (1962).
10. MARINI-SCOTTI, M. *Farmaco* (*Pavia*), *Ed. Prat.* **18**, 332 (1963).
11. HÜTTENRAUCH, R. and KLOTZ, L., *J. Chromatog.* **12**, 464 (1963).
12. ALESSANDRO, G., DALBROLLO, F., and MECARELLI, E., *Boll. Chim. Farm.* **102**, 161 (1963).
13. GSTIRNER, F. and BAVEJA, S. K., *Mitt. Deut. Pharm. Ges.* **35**, 29 (in *Arch. Pharm.* **298**, Heft 2, 1965).
14. KLOTZ, L., *Pharm. Zentralhalle* **104**, 393 (1965).
15. MORA, G. A., *Quim. Ind.* (*Bilbao*) **12**, 141 (1965).
16. PETRANGELI, B., *Boll. Chim. Farm.* **105**, 770 (1966).
17. PEKEL, N. D. and BEREZOVSKII, V. M., *Med. Prom. SSSR* **20**, 21 (1966); *Chem. Abs.* **66**, 11049 (1967).

CHAPTER 11

POLAROGRAPHY

STRICTLY speaking this method is not purely physical but is accompanied by the chemical change of reduction. It is, however, convenient to classify it separately. Methods based on the polarographic reduction of other groups in the cyano compound are given in Chapter 4 (for example, the determination of azobisisobutyronitrile, where the azo group undergoes reduction).

Most of the polarographic analytical methods are for acrylonitrile: this includes studies on pure solutions and also analyses of industrial products and residues from polymerisation procedures.

Aqueous alcohols have been the solvents principally used in polarographic analyses; lithium or quaternary ammonium salts have served as electrolyte.

The mechanism of polarographic reduction of nitriles has been studied under various conditions (pH, solvents, electrolytes). It evidently depends on these conditions and frequently radicals and anion radicals have been proposed as intermediates. Wawzonek and Pietrzyk[1] state that one-electron processes yielding anion radicals are common in certain solvents such as dimethylformamide and acetonitrile.

Thus Bargain[2] quotes one-electron reductions of many α,β-unsaturated nitriles in dimethylformamide. Finkel'shtein and Klyaev[3] consider that acrylonitrile is irreversibly reduced with the addition of one electron and one proton to yield the radical $\cdot CH_2—CH_2—CN$ which then dimerises to adiponitrile. Sevast'yanova and Tomilov[4] also assume that free radicals are formed on polarographic reduction of α,β-unsaturated nitriles, ultimately leading to a dianion; this reacts further to give the saturated nitrile or a dimer (11.1).

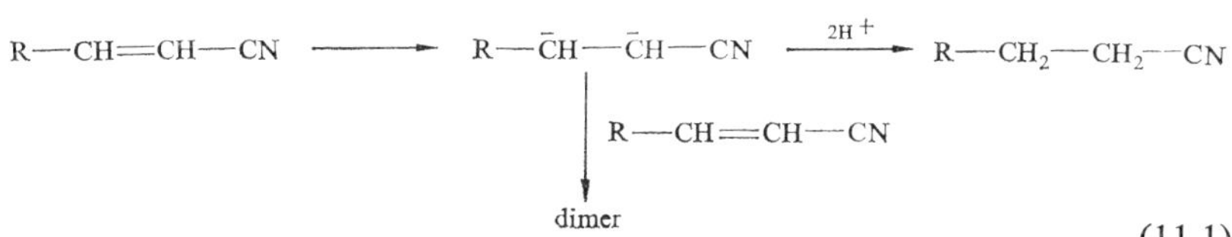

(11.1)

Platonova[5] and Gorokhovskaya and Geller[6] give reduction mechanisms for acrylonitrile in which propionitrile is the end-product.

Reiger *et al.*[7] have studied the polarographic reduction of aromatic nitriles, chiefly in dimethylformamide with tetrapropylammonium perchlorate as supporting electrolyte, and refer to one-electron reductions. Phthalonitrile, for example, gives two reduction waves corresponding to the formation of, first, the anion radical (11.2) and then the dianion (11.3) which then takes a proton from the solvent (SH), yielding benzonitrile (11.4). Zweig[8] also found two waves for pyromellitonitrile-

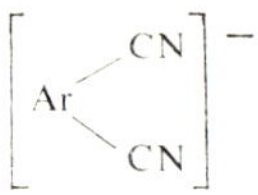

(11.2)

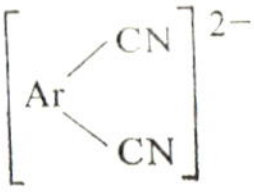

(11.3)

$$\xrightarrow{SH} Ar{-}CN + S^- + CN^- \qquad (11.4)$$

(1,2,4,5-tetracyanobenzene) in acetonitrile, at −0·66 and −1·63 volts, the former corresponding to a one-electron reduction.

The Czechoslovak school associated with Volke and with Zuman have investigated the pH-dependence of polarographic reduction of aromatic and heterocyclic nitriles. Thus Volke and co-workers[9, 10] found that both 2- and 4-cyanopyridine undergo four-electron reduction in more acid solution (Britton–Marshall buffer, pH 2·2), established later by infrared studies and preparative electrolysis as eqn. (11.5).

$$-CN + 4\varepsilon + 4H^+ \longrightarrow -CH_2{-}NH_2 \qquad (11.5)$$

The wave-height diminishes with increasing pH-value and is that of a two-electron wave at pH 10·5; this reduction is as shown in eqn. (11.6).

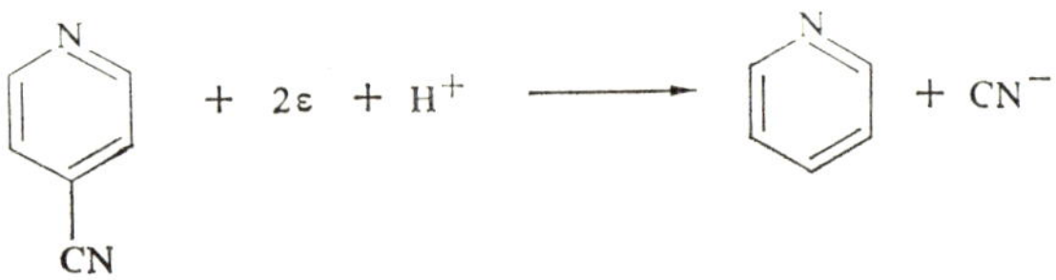

(11.6)

Manoušek and Zuman[11] studied the polarographic reduction of substituted benzonitriles at different pH-values. At above 1·5, $CN^{(-)}$ ions were likewise liberated. Even compounds containing the ketone group were preferentially reduced in this way, rather than at the ketonic carbonyl group (11.7).

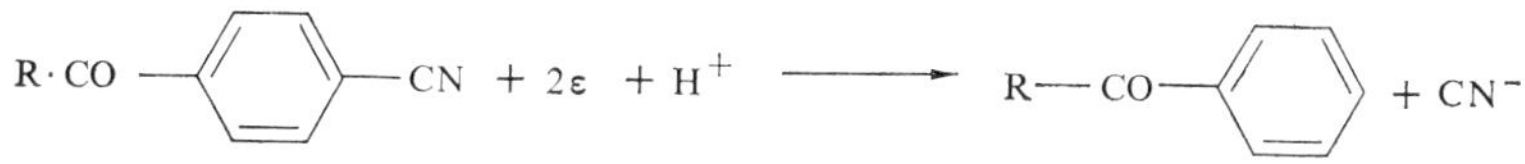

(11.7)

In more strongly acid solution (dilute sulphuric acid), the four-electron reduction of the cyano group took place.

Table 11.1 contains examples of analytical application:

TABLE 11.1. ANALYTICAL APPLICATIONS OF POLAROGRAPHY

Sample	Solution	Half-wave potential	Reference
Acrylonitrile	Water–$(CH_3)_4NI$	−2·05 volts/saturated calomel	12
Methacrylonitrile; (acrylonitrile also)	Water–$(CH_3)_4NBr$	−2·07 volts/saturated calomel; −2·02 volts/Hg anode pool	13
Acrylonitrile	50% ethanol–LiCl	−2·1 volts/standard calomel	14
Acrylonitrile	$(CH_3)_4N^{(+)}$ and $(C_4H_9)_4N^{(+)}$ electrolytes	−2·14 volts/standard calomel	15
Acrylonitrile in presence of $S_2O_8^{(2-)}$, HCN, HCHO, and other oxidation products of acrolein	$+(C_2H_5)_4NI$ + hydroquinone to prevent oxidation or polymerisation (modification of method of ref. 12)		16
2-Cyanopyridine	50% ethanol–KH_2PO_4 buffer of pH 5·6 – 7·4 (best at 5·6)	−1·35 volts/saturated calomel (pH 5·6)	17
Acrylonitrile	Aqueous alcohol–$(C_2H_5)_4NCl$	−2·05 volts	18
Acrylonitrile (control of polymerisation process)	$+(C_2H_5)_4NCl$	Polarographed between −1·9 and −2·2 volts	19

TABLE 11.1.—*cont.*

Sample	Solution	Half-wave potential	Reference
Acrylonitrile in aqueous industrial streams after separation by azeotropic distillation	$+(CH_3)_4I$; (method of ref. 12)		20
Various α,β-unsaturated nitriles, e.g. acrylo-, methacrylonitriles; dinitriles, such as of fumaric and phthalic acids	Water or 50% aqueous ethanol–Li chloride or citrate or R_4N^+ halides	Values between −1·48 and −2·37volts	21
Cinnamonitrile, α-phenyl-cinnamonitrile, fumaro-nitrile	50–75% ethanol–LiCl	−1·95, −1·85, and 2 waves, −1·30 and −2·2, respectively	22
Acrylonitrile in study of some plastic masses	10% methanol–$(CH_3)_4NI$	−2·08 volts	23
Residual acrylonitrile in polymeric systems	95% dimethylform-amide–$(nC_4H_9)_4NI$	−1·63 volts–Hg anode pool	24
Acrylonitrile in effluents from synthetic rubber plants	Neutralised, hydro-quinone added to stabilise, and distilled to separate from NH_4^+ and Na^+; then method of ref. 12		25
2-Cyanocyclopentanone (and cyclopentanone) as impurities in adiponitrile	+isopropanol–$(C_2H_5)_4NI$	−2·0 and −2·6 volts	26
Acrylonitrile in air			27
Acrylonitrile	Dimethylformamide–$(CH_3)_4NI$	−1·72 volts	6
Acrylonitrile (and acetaldehyde)	$+(CH_3)_4NI$	−1·95 to −2·0 volts and −1·8 to −1·9 volts/saturated calomel, respectively	28
Various unsaturated nitriles such as substituted acrylonitriles and dicyanobutenes	Water or dimethyl-formamide–LiCl or $(C_2H_5)_4NI$; DMF–$(C_2H_5)_4NI$ best for quantitative determination	Values between −1·36 and −2·05 volts	4
Acrylonitrile in air	Aqueous alcohol–$(C_2H_5)_4NI$	From −1·6 to 2·2 volts	29
α-Aminonitriles	$+R_4N^{(+)}$ salts		

TABLE 11.1.—*cont.*

Sample	Solution	Half-wave potential	Reference
Residual acrylonitrile in copolymers with styrene	Dry dimethylformamide–$(C_4H_9)_4NI$	From −1·7 volts	31
Acrylonitrile monomer in food packaging polymer materials, isolated by azeotropic distillation with methanol	$+(CH_3)_4NI$ to aqueous alcoholic solution	From −1·8 volts	32
Acrylonitrile in toxicological investigations of biological material	Dimethylformamide–$(C_4H_9)_4NI$	−1·63 volts/Hg pool anode	33
Iso- and terephthalonitriles	Water–LiCl	−1·84 volts; −1·62 and −1·93 volts.	34
		Terephthalonitrile determination based on −1·62 volts; both at *ca.* − 1·9 volts	35
Acrylonitrile monomer in copolymers with vinyl acetate or others	Water–$(C_2H_5)_4NI$		36
Acrylonitrile in industrial solutions	$+(C_2H_5)_4NOH$	−1·91 volts	37
Iso- and terephthalonitriles; 3- and 4-cyanobenzylamine, in m- or p-xylylenediamine	Dimethylformamide + 5% water; 0·1M $(C_2H_5)_4NI$	From −1 to −3 volts. Half-wave potentials are, respectively, −1·8 to −1·9; −1·6 to −1·7 and −2.4 to −2·6 (second wave); −2·4 to −2·6; and −2·4 to −2·6 volts	38

References

1. WAWZONEK, S. and PIETRZYK, D. J., *Anal. Chem.* **36**, 224R (1964).
2. BARGAIN, M., *Comptes Rendus* **255**, 1948 (1962); also **256**, 1990 (1963).
3. FINKEL'SHTEIN, A. V. and KLYAEV, K. I., *Tr. Sibirsk. Tekhnol. Inst.* no. 36, 106 (1963); *Chem. Abs.* **61**, 12955 (1964).
4. SEVAST'YANOVA, I. G. and TOMILOV, A. P., *Zh. Obshch. Khim.* **33**, 2815 (1963).
5. PLATONOVA, M. N., *Zh. Anal. Khim.* **11**, 310 (1956).
6. GOROKHOVSKAYA, A. S. and GELLER, B. E., *Zavod. Lab.* **28**, 809 (1962).

7. RIEGER, R. H., BERNAL, I., REINMUTH, W. H., and FRAENKEL, G. K., *J. Am. Chem. Soc.* **85**, 683 (1963).
8. ZWEIG, A., LEHNSEN, J. E., HODGSON, W. G., and JURA, W. H., *J. Am. Chem. Soc.* **85**, 3937 (1963).
9. VOLKE, J., KUBÍČEK, R., and ŠANTAVÝ, F., *Coll. Czech. Chem. Commun.* **25**, 1510 (1960).
10. VOLKE, J. and HOLUBEK, J., *Coll. Czech. Chem. Commun.* **28**, 1597 (1963).
11. MANOUŠEK, O. and ZUMAN, P., *Chem. Communs.* (*London*) 158 (1965).
12. BIRD, W. L. and HALE, C. H., *Anal. Chem.* **24**, 586 (1952).
13. SPILLANE, L. J., *Anal. Chem.* **24**, 587 (1952).
14. RYABOV, A. V. and PANOVA, G. D., *Dokl. Akad. Nauk SSSR* **99**, 547 (1954).
15. USAMI, S., *Japan Analyst* (*Bunseki Kagaku*) **4**, 424 (1955).
16. STRAUSE, S. F. and DYER, E., *Anal. Chem.* **27**, 1906 (1955).
17. DYER, E., PICKETT, O. A., STRAUSE, S. F., and WORRALL, H. E., *J. Am. Chem. Soc.* **78**, 3384 (1956).
18. JARVIE, J. M. S., OSTERYOUNG, R. A., and JANZ, G. J., *Anal. Chem.* **28**, 264 (1956).
19. PLATONOVA, M. N., *Zavod. Lab.* **23**, 539 (1957).
20. DAUES, G. W. and HAMNER, W. F., *Anal. Chem.* **29**, 1035 (1957).
21. BOBROVA, M. I. and MATVEEVA, A. N., *Zh. Obshch. Khim.* **27**, 1137 (1957).
22. BOBROVA, M. I., and MATVEEVA-KUDASHEVA, A. N., *Zh. Obshch. Khim.* **28**, 2929 (1958).
23. BEZUGLYI, V. D. and DMITRIEVA, V. N., *Zavod. Lab.* **24**, 941 (1958).
24. CLAVER, G. C. and MURPHY, M. E., *Anal. Chem.* **31**, 1682 (1959).
25. RUZICKA, O., *Vodni Hospodařstvi* **9** No. 7, 302 (1959).
26. KALUGIN, A. A., PEREPLITCHIKOVA, E. M., ZIL'BERMAN, E. N., VODZINSKII, YU. V., and KULIKOV, A. E., *Zh. Anal. Khim.* **15**, 739 (1960).
27. BERCK, B., *J. Agr. Food Chem.* **10**, 158 (1962).
28. KLYAEV, V. I., SLISARENKO, F. A., and FINKEL'SHTEIN, A. V., *Zh. Anal. Khim.* **18**, 999 (1963); *Zavod. Lab.* **30**, 160 (1964); *Ref. Zh. Khim. Abs. No.* 2G156 (1968) in *Chem. Abs.* **69**, 6018 (1968).
29. ROGACZEWSKA, T., *Chem. Anal.* (*Warsaw*) **9**, 417 (1964).
30. ZUMAN, P., MANOUŠEK, O., and HORÁK, V., *Coll. Czech. Chem. Commun.* **29**, 2906 (1965).
31. CROMPTON, T. R. and BUCKLEY, D., *Analyst* (*London*) **90**, 76 (1965).
32. CROMPTON, T. R., *Analyst* (*London*) **90**, 165 (1965).
33. THIEDE, H. and FRANZEN, E., *Wiss. Z. Martin Luther Univ. Halle-Wittenberg, Math.-Nat. Reihe* **14**, 177 (1965).
34. MEKHTIEV, S. D., SHARIFOVA, S. M., SMIRNOVA, V. P., BABAEVA, N. L., and MAMEDOVA, S. F., *Azerb. Khim. Zh.* 6 (1965); *Chem. Abs.* **64**, 14967 (1966).
35. MEKHTEV, S. D., SALIMOV, M. I., SHARIFOVA, S. M., AGAEVA, E. A. and BABAEVA, N. L., *Dokl. Akad. Nauk Azerb. SSR* **23**, 22 (1967); *Chem. Abs.* **68**, 871 (1968).
36. CHAO, L.-S. and CH'EN, S.-S. *Hua Hsuen Tung Pao* 47 (1966); *Chem. Abs.* **65**, 10669 (1966).
37. SEVAST'YANOVA, I. G., TOMILOV, A. P., and YAMALEEV, I. YA., *Zavod. Lab.* **32**, 1210 (1966).
38. ARGOVA, T. B., VESHOVA, L. V., and KARLIK, V. M., *Zavod. Lab.* **35**, 790 (1969).

CHAPTER 12

AZEOTROPIC DISTILLATION

THIS principle for the separation of nitriles has been applied only to acrylonitrile. Thus Daues and Hamner(1) separated small amounts of acrylonitrile in aqueous industrial streams by azeotropic distillation with methanol; the azeotrope contains 38·7% nitrile and boils at 61·4°. The nitrile was subsequently determined polarographically. Crompton(2) likewise used azeotropic distillation with methanol in order to isolate acrylonitrile before polarographic determination. His aim was evaluation of traces of acrylonitrile monomer in liquid extractants (such as liquid paraffin and n-heptane and also 50% ethanol, dilute HCl and Na_2CO_3) used in assessing the suitability of styrene–acrylonitrile copolymers as food packaging materials; the nitrile was first extracted from the paraffin and heptane with water and the aqueous HCl and Na_2CO_3 solutions largely neutralised; these solutions were then subjected to the distillation. Štěpánek *et al.*(3) separated traces of acrylonitrile by azeotropic distillation with isopropanol; this azeotrope contains 56% nitrile and has b.p. 71·7°. Thiede and Franzen(4) separated acrylonitrile from biological material also by distillation with isopropanol. Tweet and Miller(5) isolated ethyl acrylate and also acrylonitrile as residual monomers in polymer emulsions by rapid distillation with toluene. The acrylate and nitrile were considered to be in the first 3 ml of distillate, which was used for quantitative determination through GC. Toluene does not appear to form an azeotrope with acrylonitrile (Horsley(6) gives no data for this pair).

It is perhaps surprising that more use has not been made of this separation and purification procedure. Hydroxyl compounds yield azeotropes with high percentages of nitriles. Thus acetonitrile is present in 81, 44, 72, and 45 weight % amounts in the azeotropes with methanol, ethanol, n-propanol, and isopropanol, respectively(6). Values for acrylonitrile are given above. Butyronitrile is present in over 25% by weight in the azeotrope with n-propanol, and benzonitrile in 49% amount with *o*-cresol. Water is even more favourable and the percentages by weight of nitriles in their azeotrope with water are 85, 76, 69, 77, and 88 for aceto-, propiono-, butyro-, isobutyro-, and acrylonitrile, respectively.[6]

References

1. DAUES, G. W. and HAMNER, W. F., *Anal. Chem.* **29**, 1035 (1957).
2. CROMPTON, T. R., *Analyst (London)* **90**, 165 (1965).
3. ŠTĚPÁNEK, J. M., ČERNÁ, V. M., and PATKOVÁ, V. J., *Analyst (London)* **84**, 65 (1959).
4. THIEDE, H. and FRANZEN, E., *Wiss. Z. Martin Luther Univ. Halle-Wittenberg, Math.-Nat. Reihe* **14**, 177 (1965).
5. TWEET, O. and MILLER, W. K., *Anal. Chem.* **35**, 852 (1963).
6. HORSLEY, L. H., *Ind. Eng. Chem., Anal. Ed.* **19**, 508; *Anal. Chem.* **21**, 831 (1949).

AUTHOR INDEX

SUBJECT INDEX